RENAL DIET COOKBOOK

Essential Nutrition Guide To Manage And Improve Kidney Disease

Laurel Stevens

Copyright © 2019 Laurel Stevens

All rights reserved. No part of this publication may be reproduced, distributed, or transmitted in any form or by any means, including photocopying, recording, or other electronic or mechanical methods, without the prior written permission of the publisher, except in the case of brief quotations embodied in critical reviews and certain other noncommercial uses permitted by copyright law.

ISBN: 9781797060156

INTRODUCTION

    What Do You Know About Your kidneys?

    Function Of The Kidney

    What is kidney disease?

        What is a Dialysis?

        What is kidney transplantation?

    What causes kidney disease?

        Types of Kidney Disease

    What are the symptoms of chronic kidney disease?

    Diagnosis and Tests

Management and treatment

Renal Diet Basics

    Top Food Choices with their SODIUM contents for a Kidney Diet

    Food Choices with their Phosphorus contents for a Kidney Diet

    Top Food Choices with their potassium contents for a Kidney Diet

KIDNEY HEALTHY RECIPES

BREAKFAST RECIPES

    Low Sodium Macaroni and Cheese

    Oven Baked Apple Onion Omelet

    Quick Homemade Sausage

    Mexican Egg With Tortilla

    Eggs Burritos and Mexican Sausage Breakfast

    Spicy Breakfast Burritos

    Chicken Sandwich With Orange Salad

    Authentic Chili Rellenos Casserole

    Pumpkin Spice Applesauce Bread

    Strawberry Vanilla Bars

    Fancy Breakfast Quiche

Quick Buttermilk Pancakes

SMOOTHIE AND DRINKS

- Chocolate Cinnamon Smoothie
- Raspberry Peach Smoothie
- Spicy pineapple Smoothie
- Creamy Berry Smoothie
- Apple Beet Blend
- Lemon With Cucumber Flavored Water
- Flavored Smoothie
- Mixed Green Juice
- Smoothie Fruity
- Oatmeal Banana Shake

FISH AND SEAFOOD

- Spicy Fruit Tilapia
- Cooked Salmon Steaks
- Onion Dilled Fish
- Grilled Salmon Salsa
- Shrimp With Spaghetti
- Garnished Tortilla Pizza
- Rice Tuna Casserole
- Cooked BBQ Shrimp
- Extra Spicy Fried Fish
- Tuna Worcestershire Loaf

POULTRY AND MEAT

- Cream Cider Chicken
- Dijon Chicken Breast
- Roast Chicken with Herbs
- Cheesy Basil Chicken

- Turkey Sliders with Aioli Mixture
- Grilled Garlic Lemon Chicken Kebabs
- Broccoli Turkey Casserole
- Starter Chicken Tacos
- Herb Coated Bread Chicken
- Honey Vinegar Molasses Pork

SOUP AND STEW

- Corn Celery and Fennel Soup
- Sea Coast Roasted Red Pepper Soup
- Low Sodium White Sauce
- Chicken With Mushrooms Soup
- Beef Veggie Barley Soup
- Fancy Chili
- Piecrust Chicken Stew
- Seasoned Chicken and Gnocchi
- Creamy Potato Soup
- Rice And Chicken Carrot Soup

SALAD RECIPES

- Low Protein Strawberry Salad
- Rice Vinegar Cucumber Salad
- Creamy Pickles Pasta Salad
- Roasted Peanuts Salad with Chili-Lime Sauce
- Persimmon Pomegranate Salad
- Green molasses Salad
- Toasted Almond Summer Salad
- Lemon tarragon Orzo Salad
- Pear And wine vinegar Arugula Salad
- Asian Apple With sesame seeds Slaw

VEGETARIAN AND VEGETABLES

- Roasted Brussels sprouts
- Homemade Herb Rolls
- Lemon Cream Chess Pie
- Macaroni & Cheese In A Flash
- Blasted Cheese Garnished Vegetables
- Pinto Beans And Parslied Onions
- Lemony Roasted Asparagus
- Blasted Garlic Parsnips
- Roasted Sweet Onion And Green Beans

DESSERT RECIPES

- Tibret Sorbet
- Blueberry vanilla Bran Muffins
- Blueberry Glazed Citrus Cake Compote
- Roasted pear With Honey
- Apple Caramel Pound Cake
- Simple Lemon Curd
- Peach with Whipped Cream And Lemon
- Molded Popcorn Balls
- Pumpkin Spice Mousse Pie
- Crocked Pot Pina Cherry Cake

SIDE AND SNACKS

- Orange Chocolate Cookies
- Honey Cornmeal Muffins
- Dilled Vinegar Carrots
- Dried Cranberries With Green Beans Hazelnuts
- Toasted bread with Goat Cheese And Green Tomatoes
- Mixed Bread Pudding

- Simple Chipotle Wings
- Pineapple cabbage Coleslaw
- Refreshing Energy Bars

STAPLES
- All Purpose Herb Blend
- Cajun Seasoning
- Basil Garlic-Herb Seasoning
- Simple Low Sodium Soy Sauce
- Sarah's BBQ Sauce
- Easy Poultry Seasoning
- Mustard Red Chili Vinegar
- Mixed Mexican Blend
- Fajita Flavored Marinade
- Homemade Mushroom Broth

Common Measuring units

INTRODUCTION

Kidney disease rank among one of the leading cause of death in the United States. About 27 million American adults suffers from Kidney disease while the rate of kidney disease in children is very low, almost nothing at all. For every 70,000 children below the age of 20, only one might experience kidney disease.

A kidney disease is a situation when the kidney has been damaged and can no more perform its function properly. When you have kidney disease over a long period, and you allow the situation gets worsen, it can lead to chronic kidney disease (CKD) or kidney failure. A dialysis would be one of the options or an option of a kidney transplant.

Diet is a very important aspect of treatment for kidney disease and the impact can help you slow down the progression rate. Following a kidney diet may delay total kidney failure and also bolster kidney function. It is very important to follow a good eating and healthy lifestyle if you have kidney disease, such as monitoring the consumption of sodium, phosphorus and potassium especially.

This book provides patients with broad information and a better understanding of the importance and function of the kidney. Causes of kidney failure, kidney diseases and diet information such as dairy choice with low phosphorus, food low in sodium, fruit with low potassium and many more.

As an expert in this field, with a vast number of kidney disease patient and other patient battling with different health I have worked with, I am sure you will find a lot of useful information in this book. Countless number of kidney disease patient have been able to manage the physical symptoms and also deal with the emotional stress the consciousness can bring. This is my professional advice. Respond quickly to treating your kidney at the early stage of kidney disease and make changes to your eating lifestyle.

What Do You Know About Your kidneys?

The kidneys are those two bean-shaped organs, each about the size of a fist, located
on either side of your spine, toward your back, just below the rib cage.

What makes the Kidneys So Important?

The kidneys perform several function, among which are, the filtering of wastes and extra water from the body through passing out of urine. The kidney also produce hormone that assist in the control of calcium metabolism and maintain blood pressure (erythropoietin, renin, and calcitriol), by producing life-sustaining chemicals. It also produce hormone that stimulates red blood cell production and keep your bones healthy and strong. These steps are crucial in maintaining a stable and balance body chemicals.

In each kidney, there are about a million filtering units called nephrons, they are responsible for filtering the blood through "glomerulus". The glomerulus is a small blood vessel that function to filters the blood, and a tube-shaped structure (tubule) give back needed substances to your blood and get rid of waste.

A healthy and functioning kidney filters out about 200 quarts of blood per day, removes any excess water and the finished work is the urine we excrete. The urine is transported from the kidney to the bladder through the ureters.

Function Of The Kidney

Discharge hormones that balance blood pressure
Manufacture an create a form of vitamin D that improve strong and healthy bones
Regulate the manufacture of red blood cells
Regulate the body's fluids
Get rid of waste products from the body
Get rid of drugs from the body

What is kidney disease?

About 26 million American adults suffers from Kidney disease. A kidney disease is a situation when the kidney has been damaged and can no more perform its function properly. The renal function as it's sometimes referred to, describe the functioning state of the kidney. If both kidney organs are functioning well, a person is said to have a 100% kidney function. A person can live without noticing even if the kidney function declines to 30% or 40%. One can live normally with just one healthy kidney.

But when the kidney function decline below 25%, there is a serious problem. And a more declining in the function to about 15% to 10% means the kidney is in critical state. A dialysis would be one of the options or an option of a kidney transplant.

What is a Dialysis?

Dialysis is treatment procedure that filters toxins, excess water and solutes from the blood in people whose kidneys can no longer carry out these functions naturally, using the help of a machine. Dialysis cannot cure kidney disease, but it can increase life span. There are 2 major types of dialysis.

Hemodialysis

This is substitute for extracorporeal separation of blood product such as plasma or cells is apheresis. Hemodialysis, uses a dialysis equipment and a unique filter called a dialyzer or an artificial kidney, they are used to clean your blood of waste products, excess water, and excess salt.

Peritoneal dialysis

This is a way to remove waste products from your blood when your kidneys can no more carry out its function adequately.

In peritoneal dialysis, the dialysis solution is introduced into the patient's abdomen. A cleansing fluid captures and filters waste products from your blood then is removed through a tube (catheter).

What is kidney transplantation?
Kidney transplantation is an option of replacing a bad kidney for a healthy and functional one; so that it can filters toxins, excess water and solutes from the blood. This is done by two major ways, a deceased or living donors.

Deceased donor kidneys are gotten from people who are already dead but have agreed to give their kidneys out before their death. There is usually a sign document called organ donor cards. All kidney donations are being screened very carefully, making sure not to transmit any disease and also to have a good match. Living donors are gotten from a spouses or immediate family members. Since one can live well with just a healthy kidney.

What causes kidney disease?
A kidney disease is a situation when the kidney has been damaged and can no more perform its function properly. Kidney diseases occur when the nephrons cannot filter the blood because they are damaged. The damage can be a quick one, let's say when it's caused by toxins or injury. But mostly kidney damage occur over a period of time.

Diabetes and hypertension (High blood pressure) are two of the most common causes of the increasing kind of damage to the nephrons. When you have kidney disease over a period of time and it gets worsen, it can lead to kidney failure chronic kidney disease (CKD). Also referred to as chronic renal insufficiency.

Types of Kidney Disease

Chronic kidney disease
This is a common type of kidney disease. Chronic kidney disease or chronic renal insufficiency describes the gradual or a progressive loss of kidney function over a long period of time. It is commonly caused by diabetes and high blood pressure.

Polycystic kidney disease

Polycystic kidney disease is a genetic problem caused by one or more abnormalities formed in the genome that causes multiple cysts (a yellowish to white, oily fluid) to occur in the kidneys. These cysts can disturb the function of the kidney and provoke kidney failure. It's necessary to understand that single kidney cysts are rarely common and do not have any significant problems. Polycystic kidney disease is a more serious and separate condition.

Kidney stones
Kidney stones is also a widely known kidney problem. This is a situation where some substance and other mineral properties in the blood obstruct the kidneys, forming
solid masses (stones). During urination, kidney stones are usually being excreted, they are not very painful though and hardly lead to any significant problems.

Glomerulonephritis
Glomerulonephritis is worsening of a situation of the glomeruli. Glomeruli are tiny little structures located in the kidneys which helps to filter blood. Glomerulonephritis can be a result of drugs, infections, or congenital abnormalities (are also known as birth defects, are conditions present from birth). Mostly gets improves on its own.

What are the symptoms of chronic kidney disease?
Kidney disease is a condition that can easily go unnoticed until the disease worsens, symptoms may include:

Unexplained shortness of breath
Darkness of skin or dry, scaly skin
Puffiness around the eyes in the morning
Muscle cramping
Loss of appetite
Trouble sleeping
Difficulty concentrating
Coma
Swollen feet/ankles

Confusion
Fatigue
Excessive drowsiness or fatigue
Frequent urination, especially late at night
Pain or pressure in your chest
Anemia (a decrease in red blood cells)
Decreased sex drive
Persistent nausea

Diagnosis and Tests

How is kidney disease diagnosed?
Kidney disease can be discovered by your doctor through a routine check of your urine and blood. Three major test are recommended to ascertain a kidney disease according to the National Kidney Foundation.
1. Measuring blood pressure level may point out to a possible kidney disease.
2. ACR, this is urine test to see how much albumin (a type of protein) is in your urine. Too much of protein present in your urine might be as a result of your kidney's filtering units being damaged by disease.
3. Measuring serum creatinine helps in calculating glomerular filtration rate (GFR).
If there are any indication of kidney disease after carrying out these test, your doctor may request additional testing. Such as imaging tests, which includes computerized tomography (CT) scans, magnetic resonance imaging (MRI) and ultrasound.

An additional biopsy test call also be carried out. This is carried out by inserting a needle into the kidney to retrieve kidney tissue, an anesthesia will be given though to reduce the pain.

Management and treatment
How is chronic kidney disease treated?

There is no cure for chronic kidney disease. To treat kidney disease doctors are more focus on controlling what root cause of the disease is, they try to help you manage your cholesterol levels, blood sugar and blood level. These few steps may also be taken in early CKD to preserve an increased level of kidney function for an extended period of time:

Keeping a regular appointment with your doctor: a kidney specialist (nephrologist) may be recommended.
Quit smoking and limit alcohol
Treat anemia if present
Keep blood sugar under control.
Avoid taking painkillers and other medications that can put the kidney at risk.
Consult a dietitian about starting a heart-healthy diet that includes whole grain, fresh fruits, low-fat dairy products and veggies. This also include cutting back on protein. Eating to reduce blood cholesterol levels, and limiting potassium and sodium (salt) intake.
Cut back on foods high in cholesterol
People with a more severe kidney condition may consider the option of a dialysis and kidney transplantation.

Who is at risk for chronic kidney disease?
People with diabetes.
People with high blood pressure.
People with a family history of kidney disease.
People who often use painkillers, including over-the-counter products such as aspirin and ibuprofen.

Renal Diet Basics

It is very important to follow a good eating and healthy lifestyle if you have kidney disease, such as monitoring the consumption of sodium, phosphorus and potassium especially.

Sodium

Most foods have sodium in them. Sodium is a mineral found in salt, and we use it (Salt) mostly when preparation food. It is important to note, To help manage your blood pressure, eat foods with less sodium and salt.

You should limit sodium to 1,500 to 2,300 milligrams per day. 20 percent daily Value or more means the sodium contained in the food is high.
Do not add salt on your meal when eating.
Do away with prepared or packaged food, like foods bought from the restaurants or supermarket, they often contain much salt and sodium
Avoid using salt when cooking food.
Use sodium-free seasonings, herbs, and spices, to replace salt.
Avoid foods that are high in sodium, 600mg for a complete frozen dinner.
If you must eat canned soup, only eat soups label reduced sodium – and just eat one cup – do not eat a whole can.
Do not eat nuggets, lunch meats, sausage, hot dogs, or ham.
Only eat canned "no salt added" vegetables.
Do not use these types of salts such as "seasoned" salt, onion salt or garlic salt.

Potassium

To help your muscles and nerves work optimally, Eat foods with the right amount of potassium. When blood potassium levels are too low or high, Problems can occur. It can cause a possible heart attack due to changes in the way the heart beats.
Most fruits, vegetables, meat and milk are high in Potassium, some have to be avoided and others taken in moderation.
Potassium-rich foods to avoid:
Oranges and orange juice

Winter squash
Melons such as honeydew and cantaloupe excluding watermelon
Pumpkin
Dried beans – all kinds
Tomatoes juice and tomato sauce
Prune juice
Grapefruit juice
Bananas
Potatoes can be eating in moderation, provided they are soaked in water for long hours, after cutting and peeling. Discard water and also cook in plenty water.
Cooked greens, Swiss Chard, kale, spinach, collards,

Phosphorus

Phosphorus can build up in your blood when the kidneys do not function adequately. To help protect your blood vessels and bones, choose drinks and eat foods that are low in phosphorus. For people that have Chronic Kidney Disease, phosphorus can easily build up in your blood which will cause lack of calcium in your bones. This can cause calcium to be pulled from your bones. Bone disease can make your bone weak or even break. Dairy foods are major source of phosphorus, they should be taken with caution. Reduce milk to 1 cup per day.

White bread are better than whole grain breads

Some vegetables are high in phosphorus.

Avoid these kind of drinks: tangerine pineapple, Mountain Dew, Dr. Pepper, colas, root beers, Beer Aquafina and Cool iced tea.

Top Food Choices with their SODIUM contents for a Kidney Diet

Food type serving	Average sodium amount per
Vegetables, frozen or fresh, no added salt (summer squash, eggplant, cucumbers, carrots , broccoli, asparagus)	0-85 mg (1/2 cup)
Vegetables, low- or no-salt, canned,	

(mushroom, corn, carrots, asparagus mixed vegetables) 5-35 mg (1/2 cup)

Fruit, fresh (watermelon, tangerines, pineapple, pears, lemon, peaches, cherries, berries ,apples) 0 mg (whole or 1 cup)

Seafood, dairy, poultry and meats

Food type	Average amount per serving
Skinless Chicken and grilled, no salt added	20-80 mg (3 oz)
Fish (tuna, shrimp, halibut, crab, cod, catfish,)	40-200 mg (3 oz)
Cooked Egg whites	55 mg (large)
Beef, no salt added	45-65 mg (3 oz)
Pork loin	54 mg (3 oz)

Rice, pasta and grains	
White bread	170 mg (1 slice)
Crackers, no-salt or low	0-20 mg (serving size)
Rice, white	0 mg (1 C)
Cereal, crispy or puffed	0-220 mg (1 C)

Sauces, seasonings and   condiments,

Tabasco	35 mg (1 tsp)
Mrs. Dash herb seasoning	0 mg (1/4 tsp))
Cranberry sauce	10 mg (1/4 cup)
Lemon	0 mg (whole)
Vinegar	0 mg (1 tsp)
Jam or jelly	6 mg (1 tbsp)
Mustard, yellow	56 mg (1 tsp)
Horseradish	50 mg (1 tsp))
Herbs and spices without salt	

(garlic or onion powder)	0 mg (1 tsp))
Garlic	0 mg (whole)

Food Choices with their Phosphorus contents for a Kidney Diet

Meat or Poultry	Phosphorus Content
Chicken breast, skinless	190 mg
Turkey breast meat, skinless	185 mg
Pork roast	190 mg
Lamb chop	185 mg
Beef, pot roast	155 mg
Pork chop	200 mg
Hamburger patty, 90 percent lean	170 mg
Veal chop	200 mg
Turkey thigh meat, skinless	170 mg
Chicken thigh, skinless	150 mg
Beef, sirloin steak	195 mg

Phosphorus content for a 3-ounce portion, cooked:

Seafood	Phosphorus Content
Oysters, Eastern	120 mg
Sea bass	210 mg
Mahi Mahi	155 mg
Rockfish	195 mg
Lobster	160 mg
King crab	192 mg
Shrimp	120 mg
Tuna, canned	130 mg
Snow crab	120 mg
Yellow fin tuna	210 mg
Salmon, Atlantic farmed	215 mg

Bread	Phosphorus Content (1-ounce portion)
Sourdough bread	30 mg
Pita bread, white	58 mg
Blueberry, plain, onion	53-70 mg
Italian or French bread or rolls	28-29 mg
No baking powder	
Flour tortilla	20-37 mg
White bread	25 mg
Light wheat bread	38 mg
English muffin	52-76 mg
Flat bread	48 mg
6-inch Corn tortilla	75 mg
Bagel: cinnamon raisin,	

Rice or Pasta	Phosphorus Content (1/2 cup portion, cooked)
Plain white rice, short	
Spaghetti	42 mg
Rice noodles	14-28 mg
Couscous	20 mg
Macaroni	40 mg
Long grain or medium	35 mg
Pearled barley,	43 mg
Egg noodles	50-60 mg

Dairy, Egg Whites and dairy Substitutes	Phosphorus Content (1-ounce portion unless stated otherwise)
With no calcium-phosphate	29 mg
Soy milk	50-125 mg
Almond Breeze, Almond milk, original	50 mg
Sherbet	38 mg
Sour cream, 2 tbsp	20-40 mg
Pasteurized egg whites,	15 mg

Unenriched rice milk
Non-dairy whipped topping, 2 tbsp   0-10 mg
Non-dairy creamer with no phosphate additives   40-53 mg

Snack Food	(Plus Serving Size)	Phosphorus Content
Radishes	1	9 mg
Blueberries	1/2 cup	9 mg
Fresh Pineapple	1/2 cup	6 mg
Apple	1 medium	10 mg
Peach	1 medium	10 mg
Fig bar	2 bars	10-25 mg
Popcorn, unsalted	1 cup	8 mg
Low-sodium crackers	1 ounce	20-35 mg
Fruit cocktail	1/2 cup	17 mg
Fruit candies		
Gummy or chews		0 mg
Cherries	1/2 cup	15 mg
Fresh Strawberries	1/2 cup	18 mg
Celery	1 stalk	10 mg
Pretzels, unsalted	1 ounce	20-40 mg
Baby carrots	9 pieces	25 mg
Applesauce	1/2 cup	6 mg

Cheese	(Plus Serving Size)	Phosphorus Content
Cottage cheese,	1/4 cup	92 mg
Cream cheese,	2 tbsp	20-40 mg
Blue cheese,	1 ounce	110 mg
Grated Parmesan cheese	2 tbsp	72 mg
Feta cheese,	1 ounce	96 mg
Neufchatel cheese,	1 ounce	39 mg

Top Food Choices with their potassium contents for a Kidney Diet

Food (no added salt table)	Serving size	Potassium (mg)
Tea, brewed	1 cup	90
Sugar, powdered	1 tsp /1 tbsp	0
Spaghetti, no sauce	½ cup	30
Cheese	1 oz	20-30
Raspberries	½ cup	90
Sherbet	½ cup	70
Salt	1 tsp	0
Radishes	1 radish	10
Popcorn	1 cup	20-25
Pineapple	1/2 cup	100
Olives	5 large	Less than 5
Soybean, sunflower)	1 tbsp	0
Macaroni	½ cup	65
Rice (white, brown)	½ cup	50
Lime	juice of 1 fruit	45
Applesauce	1/2 cup	90
Lettuce	1 cup	100
Tortilla, flour or corn	1	50
Lemon	1 fruit juice	50
Pork, Hot dog and beef	1	75
Beans, green	1/2 cup	90
Butter	1 Tbsp	Less than 5
Grape	9 grapes	90
Gelatin	½ cup	Less than 5
Peeled cucumber	½ cup	80
Hummus	1 Tbsp	35
Cranberry juice	½ cup	20
Cereal (puffed wheat)	1 cup	Less than 5
Cereal (puffed rice)	1 cup	15
Blueberries	½ cup	60
Bagel, plain, enriched	10 cm	70
Bread, whole grain	1 slice	60

NOTE:

Potassium: Limit your potassium intake to 2,000 milligrams per day, if you are on hemodialysis. Limit your potassium intake to 3,500 milligrams per day, if you are on short daily dialysis or peritoneal dialysis.

Phosphorus: Limit your phosphorus intake to about 1,000 milligrams per day, if you are on dialysis.

Protein: If you have kidney disease but not on dialysis, low protein diet might be beneficial. Ask your dietitian or kidney doctor for guidelines.

Sodium: Most of the recipes are low in sodium, limit your sodium intake to 1,500-2,300 milligrams per day.

KIDNEY HEALTHY RECIPES

BREAKFAST RECIPES

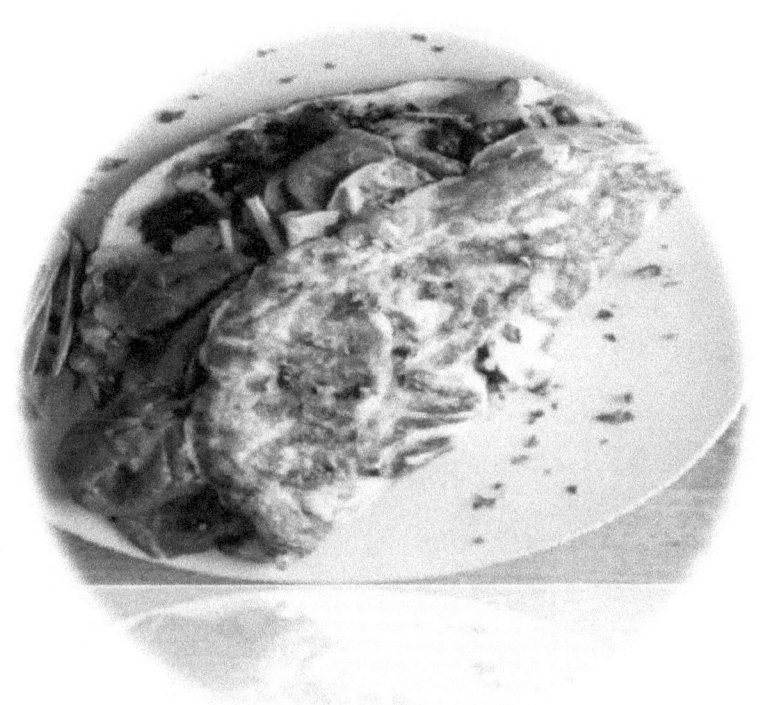

Low Sodium Macaroni and Cheese

Prep time: 5 minutes
Cook time: 5-7 minutes
Servings: 4

Ingredients:

1/4 tsp of dried mustard
1 tsp of unsalted butter or margarine
1/2 cup of cheddar cheese, grated
2 or 3 cups hot water
2 cups of any shape kind of noodles

Preparations:

1. Cook noodles in hot water for about 5-7 minutes until soft. Drain.
2. While the noodles is still hot, top with a sprinkle of cheese, stir in mustard and butter.
3. If desired, bake in oven for 10-15 minutes at 350 or until top is golden brown.

Nutrition Facts per serving

Calories	163 g
Phosphorus	138 mg
Potassium	39 mg
Sodium	114 mg
Protein	6 g
Carbohydrates	20 g

Oven Baked Apple Onion Omelet

Prep time: 12 minutes
Cook time: 15 to 18 minutes
Servings: 2

Ingredients:

2 tbsp of shredded cheddar cheese
1 large Peel and core apple, (Gala, Jonagold, or McIntosh are the best)
3/4 cup of sweet onion
1 tbsp of butter
1/8 tsp of black pepper
1 tbsp of water
1/4 cup of 1% low fat milk
3 large eggs

Preparation:

1. Heat up the oven to 400º F.
2. Slice the onion and apple thinly.
3. In a small bowl, beat together milk, eggs, pepper and water; set aside.
4. Heat butter over medium heat in a small ovenproof pan. Add apple and onion to the pan and sauté about 5 to 6 minutes or until onion is tender.
5. Evenly spread the apple mixture in the skillet and then spread egg/milk mixture into the pan and cook until the edges starts to set. Top with a sprinkle of cheddar cheese.
6. Bake in the oven, about 10 to 12 minutes or until the center is totally set.
7. Divide omelet in two and serve immediately.

Nutrition Facts per serving
Calories	284 g
Carbohydrates	22 g
Potassium	341 mg
Phosphorus	238 mg
Protein	13 g
Sodium	169 mg

Quick Homemade Sausage

Servings: 8

Ingredients:

1/4 tsp of ground red pepper

1-1/2 tsp of black pepper

1 tsp of dried, crushed basil

2 tsp of sugar or sugar substitute

2 tsp of ground sage

1 lbs of ground pork or beef or turkey

Preparation:

1. Mix together all ingredients in a large bowl.
2. Form into 8 equal patties.
3. Cook until cooked to desired degree of doneness or freeze for later use.

Nutrition Facts per serving

Calories	133 g
Carbohydrates	2 g
Potassium	171 mg
Phosphorus	98 mg
Protein	11 g
Sodium	31 mg

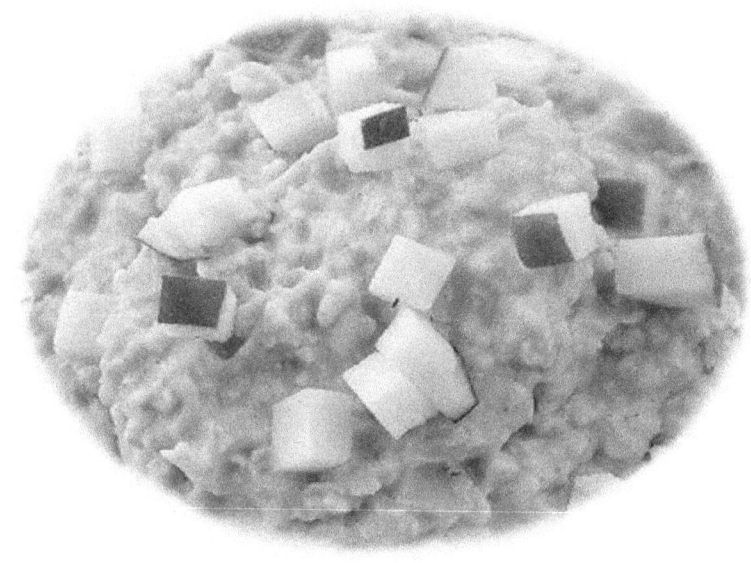

Mexican Egg With Tortilla

Prep time: 7 minutes
Cook time: 5 minutes
Servings: 6

Ingredients:
1 (6oz) bag of no salt added tortilla chips, broken up
2 Tbsp of Butter
1/4 cup of low salt ketchup
1 tsp of chili powder
2 thinly sliced green onions
8 eggs (or egg beaters)

Preparations:
1. Beat eggs in a bowl until smooth and fluffy.
2. Add the ketchup onion and chili powder and beat until nicely mixed. Set aside.
3. Heat the butter in a fry pan, add in the tortilla chips and sauté over medium high heat, for 2 to 3 minutes or until the chips have turned lightly golden.
4. Mix in egg mixture and scramble until cooked the way you desire. Serve over heated plates.

Note: You can replace unsalted tortilla chips with flour tortillas, cut into 4 and bake in the oven at 350°F until crisp.

Nutrition Facts per serving
Calories	297 g
Phosphorus	179 mg
Potassium	152 mg
Sodium	267 mg
Protein	11 g
Carbohydrates	20 g

Eggs Burritos and Mexican Sausage Breakfast

Prep time: 3 minutes
Cook time: 3-4 minutes
Servings: 6

Ingredients:
3 flour tortillas
3 beaten eggs
3 oz of Mexican sausage (chorizo)

Preparations:
1. Heat up a non-stick skillet over medium heat. Fry chorizo on each side, for about 2 to 3 minutes in the skillet until crispy and dark in color.
2. Pour in the beaten eggs and cook until done.
3. Fill chorizo egg mixture in warmed tortillas and fold up the bottom edges, then roll up, to prevent the chorizo egg filling from falling out.

Nutrition Facts per serving
Calories   320 g
Phosphorus   170 mg
Potassium   214 mg
Sodium   659 mg
Protein   16 g
Carbohydrates   18 g

Spicy Breakfast Burritos

Prep time: 5 minutes
Cook time: 10 minutes
Servings: 4

Ingredients:
4 (6-inch) corn tortillas
8 eggs, beaten
4 thinly sliced green onions (scallions)
Half diced red bell pepper
1 1/2 tsp of olive or canola oil

Preparation:
1. In a medium frying pan, heat the oil on moderate heat.
2. Add green onion and bell pepper and cook about 3 minutes until softened.
3. Add in the eggs and scramble until eggs are set, about 5 minutes.
4. Place a damp paper towels, add the tortillas and place another damp paper towels, then arrange on a plate.
5. Place the tortillas in the Microwave for 2 minutes. Fill warm tortillas with the egg mixture. Fold tortillas edges and roll up to enjoy.
If desired, add a sprinkle of chili powder or dash of hot sauce.

Nutrition Facts per serving
Calories	232 g
Phosphorus	207 mg
Potassium	211 mg
Sodium	152 mg
Protein	14 g
Carbohydrates	16 g

Chicken Sandwich With Orange Salad

Servings: 6

Ingredients:

1/3 cup of mayonnaise
1 cup of Mandarin oranges
1/4 cup nicely sliced onion
1/2 cup of chopped green pepper
1/2 cup of diced celery
1 cup of cooked chicken, chopped

Preparation:

1. Combine onion, green pepper, celery and chicken, toss to combine.
2. Add mayonnaise and mandarin oranges. Gently stir and serve on top of bread.

Nutrition Facts per serving

Calories	170 g
Phosphorus	106 mg
Potassium	241 mg
Sodium	97 mg
Protein	12 g
Carbohydrates	6 g

Authentic Chili Rellenos Casserole

Prep time: 20 minutes
Cook time: 30-40 minutes
Servings: 6

Ingredients:
1 tsp of low sodium baking powder
1 cup of flour
2/3 cup of milk
8 large eggs
8 fresh whole pasilla peppers
1 cup of ricotta cheese
6 oz of shredded jack cheese
6 oz of shredded cheddar cheese

Preparation:
1. Warm up the oven to 350 F
2. Broil peppers in the oven at 500 F until slightly charred (keep an eye on it).
Remove and cover with plastic wrap in a bowl and allow cooling for 15 minutes.
3. Remove the skins of the roasted peppers. Put ricotta and cheese in peppers and transfer into a greased 9×13 pan.
4. Beat flour, milk, baking powder and eggs in blender or food processor until smooth.
Pour over peppers evenly.
5. Place in the preheated oven and bake for 30-40 minutes.
Serve while it's hot.

Nutrition Facts per serving
Calories	273 g
Phosphorus	325 mg
Potassium	388 mg
Sodium	420 mg
Protein	24 g
Carbohydrates	22 g

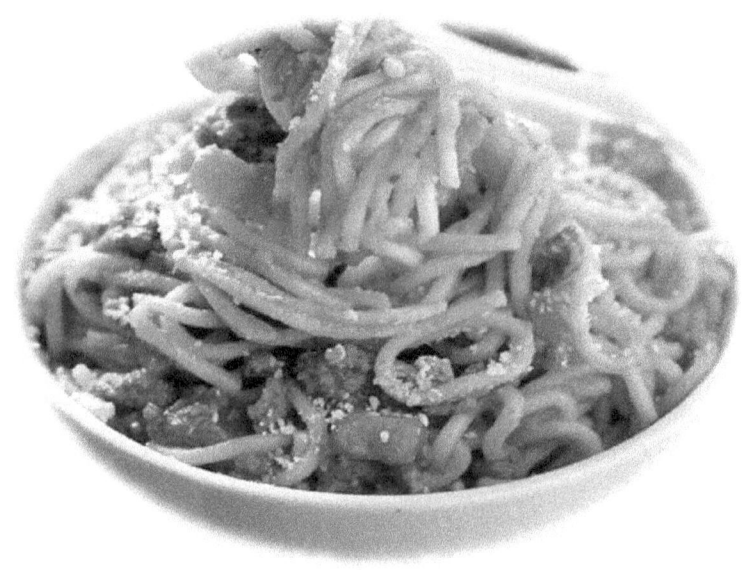

Pumpkin Spice Applesauce Bread

Prep time: 10 minutes

Cook time: varies

Servings: 12

Ingredients:

2 tsp of pumpkin pie spice

1/2 tsp of baking powder

1 tsp of baking soda

2 cups of all-purpose flour

2 eggs

1/2 cup of vegetable oil

1 cup of brown sugar

1 1/2 cups of applesauce, unsweetened

Preparation:

1. Heat up the oven to 350 F.
2. Lightly grease muffin pan or loaf pan.
3. Whisk together the applesauce, eggs, oil and brown sugar in a medium bowl.
4. Mix remaining ingredients together in a separate bowl.
5. Combine the flour mixture with applesauce mixture and stir until just combined (Be mindful not to over mix).
6. Transfer batter in the greased muffin pan or loaf pan.

7. Bake for about 20 minutes for muffins and 50-60 minutes for loaf
8. Insert a toothpick in the center to check if it's done. It's done when the toothpick comes out clean.

Nutrition Facts per serving
Calories   252 g
Phosphorus   41 mg
Potassium   82 mg
Sodium   141 mg
Protein   3 g
Carbohydrates   38 g

Strawberry Vanilla Bars

Prep time: 10 minutes
Cook time: 25-30 minutes
Servings: 24

Ingredients:
1 cup of strawberry jam
1 tsp of vanilla extract
1/4 cup of water
1 egg
1/2 cup of vegetable oil
1 tsp of baking powder
1/2 cup of sugar
2 cups of flour

Preparation:
1. Heat up the oven to 400 F.
2. Mix baking powder, flour and sugar in a mixing bowl. Mix in the vegetable oil until crumbly.
3. Add vanilla extract, egg and water, and stir well.
4. Grease a 9×13 inch pan and evenly spread 2/3 of batter in the pan and then Press.
5. Spread jam evenly over the top
6. Make flat crumbs over the top, with the remaining batter.

7. Transfer to the oven and bake for 25-30 mins. Allow to Cool in pan and slice into 24 bars.

Nutrition Facts per serving
Calories   131 g
Phosphorus   120 mg
Potassium   14 mg
Sodium   24 mg
Protein   1 g
Carbohydrates   21 g

Fancy Breakfast Quiche
Prep time: 5 minutes
Cook time: 45-60 minutes
Servings: 6
Ingredients:
4 oz of grated cheese
1 (9 inches) deep-dish frozen pie shell
2 cups of total filling (leftover meat or vegetables)
1 cup of 2% milk or lower
6 Eggs
Preparation:
1. Heat up the oven to 350 F.
2. Mix filling, milk, eggs and cheese together
3. Transfer mixture into the frozen pie shell
4. Bake about 45-60 minutes or until a knife inserted into the center comes out dry.
Let stand for 5 minutes.

Nutrition Facts per serving
Calories   131 g
Phosphorus   278 mg
Potassium   257 mg
Sodium   409 mg
Protein   1 g
Carbohydrates   21 g

Quick Buttermilk Pancakes

Prep time: 7 minutes
Cook time: 5 minutes
Servings: 9

Ingredients:

¼ cup of canola oil plus 1 tbsp for cooking
2 large eggs
2 cups low-fat buttermilk
1½ tsp of baking soda
2 tbsp of sugar
1 tsp of cream of tartar
2 cups of all-purpose flour

Preparations:

1. Heat up the skillet over medium- high heat.
2. Combine eggs, oil and buttermilk in a bowl. Add dry ingredients to the wet ingredient and whisk until completely moist.
3. Grease the skillet with 1 tablespoon of canola oil. Scoop the batter in 1/3 cup measuring cup onto the skillet, leaving 2 inches gap between pancakes.
4. Cook about 3 minutes or until bubbles form on top, then flip and cook the other side, about 2 minutes. If desired, serve with fresh berries and a side of eggs

Nutrition Facts per serving

Calories	217 g
Phosphorus	100 mg
Potassium	182 mg
Sodium	330 mg
Protein	6 g
Carbohydrates	27 g

SMOOTHIE AND DRINKS

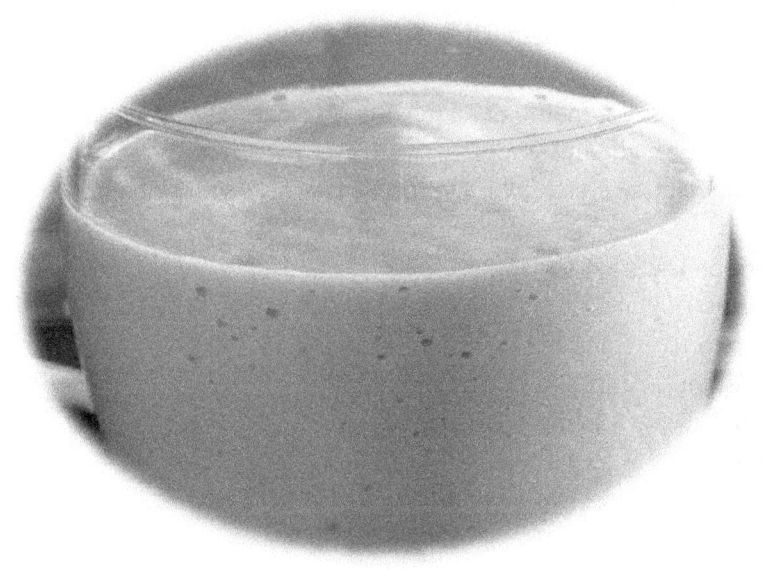

Chocolate Cinnamon Smoothie

Servings: 4

Ingredients:

Pinch of nutmeg
¼ tsp of ground cinnamon
¼ cup of condensed milk
½ cup of evaporated milk
(Optional) 2 tbsp of Southern Comfort liqueur
2 cups of ice
2 scoops of whey protein (chocolate-flavored)

Preparations:

1. Set aside the cinnamon and mix the rest ingredient in blender, about 2 minutes on high until smooth.
2. Add whipped cream over the top and garnish with cinnamon.

Nutrition Facts per serving
Calories   5 g
Phosphorus   113 mg
Potassium   252 mg
Sodium   83 mg
Protein   15 g
Carbohydrates   15 g

Raspberry Peach Smoothie

Servings: 3

Ingredients:

1 cup of unfortified almond milk
1 tbsp of honey or stevia or splenda sweetener
1/2 cup of tofu
1 medium slice peach, pit removed
1 cup of frozen raspberries

Preparations:

1. Combine all the ingredients in blender and blend until you have a smooth mixture.

Nutrition Facts per serving

Calories	12 g
Phosphorus	72 mg
Potassium	261 mg
Sodium	53 mg
Protein	6.3 g
Carbohydrates	23 g

Spicy pineapple Smoothie

Servings: 2

Ingredients:
1 pinch of red pepper flakes
1 teaspoon of Stevia
½ cup of unsweetened pineapple juice
1 (8 oz) cup of tofu, firm
1 cup of pineapple, canned or fresh

Preparations:
1. Combine all the ingredients in blender and blend until you have a smooth mixture.

Nutrition Facts per serving

Calories	189 g
Phosphorus	121 mg
Potassium	349 mg
Sodium	5 mg
Protein	13.4 g
Carbohydrates	32 g

Creamy Berry Smoothie

Servings: 2

Ingredients:

2 (13 grams) scoops of whey protein powder
4 oz of very cold water
1/2 cup of whipped cream topping
1 tsp of liquid blueberry raspberry flavor enhancer drops, (Crystal Light)
2 ice of cubes
1 cup of fresh mixed berries or frozen (blackberries, raspberries, blueberries, strawberries)

Preparation:

1. Combine all ingredient without the whipped cream and protein powder in a blender and blend until mixed well.
2. Add in the whipped cream and blend well.
3. Add whey protein powder and blend until smooth.
Serve and enjoy.

Nutrition Facts per serving
Calories	104 g
Phosphorus	49 mg
Potassium	141 mg
Sodium	15 mg
Protein	6 g
Carbohydrates	11 g

Apple Beet Blend

Servings: 2

Ingredients:

1/4 cup of parsley
1 celery stalk
1 medium fresh carrot
1/2 medium beet
1/2 medium apple

Preparation:

1. In a juicer, Process parsley, celery, carrot, beet and apple to extract juice.
2. Serve immediately or chill in the refrigerator.

Nutrition Facts per serving

Calories	53 g
Phosphorus	36 mg
Potassium	338 mg
Sodium	66 mg
Protein	1 g
Carbohydrates	13 g

Lemon With Cucumber Flavored Water

Servings: 10

Ingredients:

10 cups of water
1/4 cup of finely chopped fresh mint leaves
1/4 cup of finely chopped fresh basil leaves
1 thinly sliced lemon
1 medium thinly sliced cucumber

Preparation:

1. Combine all the ingredients into a pitcher.
2. Chill in the Refrigerator overnight before serving.

Nutrition Facts per serving

Calories	4 g
Phosphorus	4 mg
Potassium	38 mg
Sodium	8 mg
Protein	0 g

Carbohydrates   1 g

Flavored Smoothie

Servings: 2
Ingredients:
1 cup of crushed ice
1 cup of cold water
2 scoops of vanilla-flavored whey protein powder
8 oz of canned fruit cocktail, plus juice
Preparation:
1. In a blender, Mix together all the ingredients until smooth.

Nutrition Facts per serving
Calories   186 g
Phosphorus   118 mg
Potassium   282 mg
Sodium   62 mg
Protein   23 g
Carbohydrates 19 g

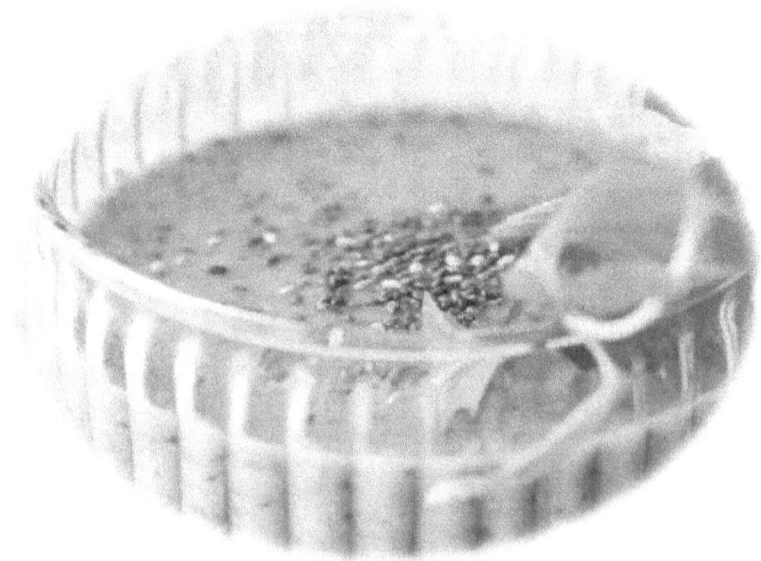

Mixed Green Juice

Ingredients:
1 medium cucumber
1/2 cup of fresh pineapple
1/2 lemon
2 medium green apples, cored

Preparation:
1. In a juicer, Process cucumber, lemon, pineapple and apples to extract juice.

Nutrition Facts per serving
Calories   130 g
Phosphorus   46 mg
Potassium   366 mg
Sodium   4 mg
Protein   1 g
Carbohydrates   31 g

Smoothie Fruity

Servings: 2 5-ounce servings

Ingredients:
3 ice cubes, crushed
1/2 cup of juice, such as cranberry, orange, grape
2 tsp of tang powder
1/2 cup of egg substitute

Preparation:
1. Blend the ingredients together in a blender until you have a smoothie mixture.
2. Add in ice cubes and blend until slushy.

Nutrition Facts per serving
Calories   87 g
Phosphorus   73 mg
Potassium   209 mg
Sodium   108 mg

Protein   7 g
Carbohydrates 9 g

Oatmeal Banana Shake

Servings: 2
Ingredients
1 1/2 tsp of vanilla extract
1 tbsp of wheat germ
1/2 of banana, frozen and cut into chunks
2 tbsp of brown sugar
1/2 cup of chilled cooked oatmeal
2/3 cup of skim milk
Preparation
1. Blend the oatmeal in blender.   Add in vanilla, banana, wheat germ, brown sugar and milk. Blend until mixture is smooth and thick. If desired, serve with ice.

Nutrition Facts per serving
Calories   172 g
Phosphorus   160 mg
Potassium   297 mg
Sodium   42 mg
Protein   6 g
Carbohydrates 33 g

FISH AND SEAFOOD

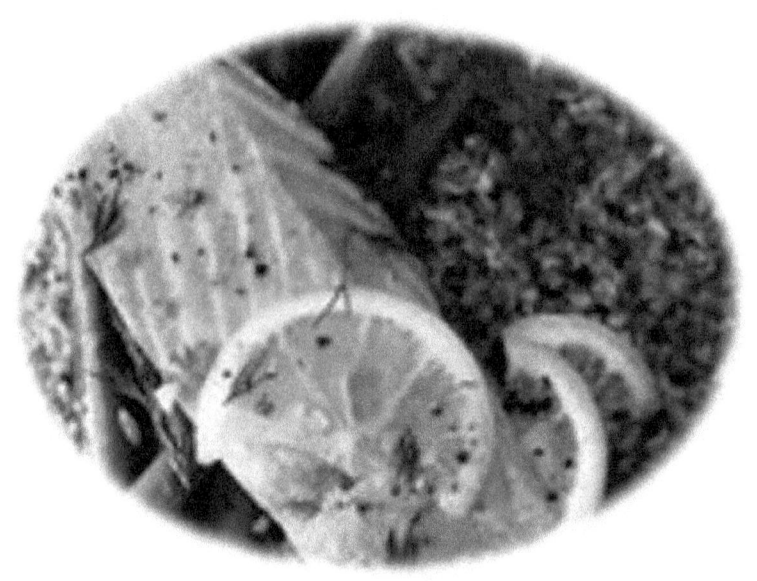

Spicy Fruit Tilapia

Prep time: 15 minutes
Cook time: 12-17 minutes
Servings: 4

Ingredients:

1 tsp of ground black pepper
4 tsp of orange juice
2 tsp of grated orange peel (zest)
½ cup of sliced green onions
¾ cup celery, julienned
1 cup of julienned carrots
16 oz of tilapia

Preparations:

Preheat oven to 450° F.

1. Mix together the orange zest, green onions, celery and carrots in a small bowl.
2. Cut the tilapia equally into four parts. Spray nonstick cooking spray on 4 large squares foil.
3. Arrange quarter vegetables over each foil piece, diverging from the exact center a bit and add the fish over the top. Sprinkle each top with 1 tsp of juice of orange. Add ground black pepper to season.
4. Fold foil and compress foil edges into small folds to make a pouch or envelope and set the foil packets onto a baking sheet.
5. Bake in the oven for about 12-17 minutes (depending on the fish thickness). Or until fish flakes easily with a fork.
6. Remove envelops or pouches and arrange over the plates. Be careful of the steam while opening.

Nutrition Facts per serving
Calories	133 g
Phosphorus	214 mg
Potassium	543 mg
Sodium	97 mg
Protein	24 g
Carbohydrates	6 g

Cooked Salmon Steaks

Prep time: 10 minutes
Cook time: 6 minutes
Servings: 4

Ingredients:
4 lemon wedges
1 tsp of paprika
1 tsp of crumbled dried tarragon
2 lemon slices, halved
4 thinly onion slices
1/2 tsp of onion powder
1/2 tsp of garlic powder
1/2 tsp of lemon pepper
1 1/2 tsp of lemon juice
4 6 oz of salmon steaks
3 tbsp of butter

Preparation:
(I use an 8×8" class baking dish)
1. Grease the dish with 1 tbsp of butter.
2. Arrange salmon in the greased dish.
3. Sprinkle with lemon pepper, lemon juice, onion powder and garlic powder, and then
Place lemon piece and 1 onion slice on top of each salmon.
4. Sprinkle with paprika and tarragon.
5. Use plastic wrap to cover salmon steak and microwave about 6 minutes on high until salmon is cooked. Serve right away with lemon wedges.

Nutrition Facts per serving
Calories   392 g
Phosphorus   504 mg
Potassium   735 mg
Sodium   150 mg
Protein   34 g
Carbohydrates 3g

Onion Dilled Fish

Prep time: 5 minutes
Cook time: 17-20 minutes
Servings: 6

Ingredients:
4 tsp of lemon juice
Dash of pepper
1/2 tsp of dill weed
1/4 tsp of mustard powder
1 tsp of instant onion, (freeze dried) minced
1 1/2 lbs or fresh, firm white fish

Preparation:
1. Warm up the oven to 475 F.
2. Rinse the fish very well and pat dry.
3. Place fish over a baking dish.
4. Combine 2 tablespoons of water, dill weed, mustard pepper and onion, add in lemon juice and spread evenly on top of the fish.
5. Bake in the oven uncovered for 17-20 minutes.

Nutrition Facts per serving
Calories   112 g
Phosphorus   194 mg
Potassium   350 mg
Sodium   63 mg
Protein   23 g
Carbohydrates   1 g

Grilled Salmon Salsa

Prep Time: 5 minutes
Cook Time: 8 mins
Servings: 4 servings per recipe

Ingredients:

1 tbsp of dried oregano
1 tbsp of onion powder
4 (6 oz each) of salmon fillets, skin on
2 tbsp of black pepper
1 tbsp of cayenne pepper
1/2 tsp of black pepper
2 tsp of creole seasoning
2 tbsp of garlic powder
2 1/2 tsp of paprika
1 tbsp of dried thyme
Fruit Salsa to taste
4 tbsp of olive oil, divided

Preparation:

1. Brush the salmon on both sides with olive oil and season with pepper and creole seasoning.
2. Arrange the skin side of the fish down on the grill and cook for 3 minutes, turn 45 degrees and cook for 3 more minutes.
3. Turn fish once more and cook about 2 minutes or until desired doneness.
4. Serve fish top with fruit salsa.

Nutrition Facts per serving

Calories	374 g
Phosphorus	419 mg
Potassium	687 mg
Sodium	410 mg
Protein	38g
Carbohydrates	3 g

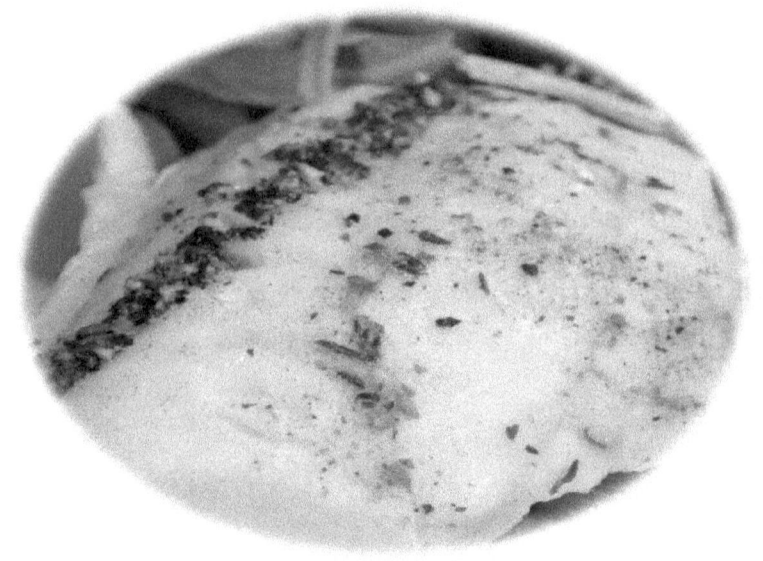

Shrimp With Spaghetti

Prep time: 10 minutes
Cook time: 10 minutes
Servings: 4

Ingredients:
1/2 pounds of spaghetti
1/3 cup of extra virgin olive oil
1/3 cup of dry white wine
2 crushed cloves garlic
1/4 teaspoon of crushed red chilies
1 diced red pepper
1 pounds of raw shrimp
1/3 cup of toasted fresh bread crumbs
Freshly ground pepper
(Optional) fresh Chopped parsley

Preparations:
1. Cook pasta the way instructed in the package instructions. Drain.

2. Heat olive oil in large skillet over high-medium heat and add red chilies and garlic. Cook and stir for 1 minute.
3. Add in the peppers and cook about 5 minutes more (do not brown).
4. Pour the shrimp and keep cooking for 1 more minute. Add the wine and reduce to medium heat. Cook until shrimp starts to curl and turns opaque. Keep warm until the spaghetti is ready.
5. Pour the shrimp sauce on pasta in a serving dish and toss with breadcrumbs until well coated. Garnish with parsley and freshly ground pepper.

Nutrition Facts per serving
Calories   716 g
Phosphorus   215 mg
Potassium   340 mg
Sodium   326 mg
Protein   28g
Carbohydrates   25 g

Garnished Tortilla Pizza

Prep time: 15 minutes
Cook time: 10 minutes
Servings: 4

Ingredients:

For the pizza:
2 flour tortillas
1/2 cup of grated mozzarella cheese
6 roughly chopped basil leaves
1/4 cup of sliced vidalia onion
8 (31/40 count) large shrimp, peeled, deveined, and remove tail

For the pesto:
1 tsp of grated parmesan cheese
1/8 tsp of ground black pepper
1 tbsp of extra virgin olive oil
1 tbsp of lemon juice
1 garlic clove
1 red pepper, roasted

Preparations:
1. Warm up the oven to 425 Degrees (conventional oven).
2. Puree pesto ingredients in a blender or food processor.
3. On a cookie sheet, place flour tortillas and cover the two tortillas surface with the roasted red pepper pesto evenly.
4. Add the basil and onions and then sprinkle the top with mozzarella cheese. Cut shrimp lengthwise in half and place over pizzas.
5. Bake about 10 minutes or until the shrimp turn pink in color, tortillas turn golden brown and crisp.

Nutrition Facts per serving
Calories   246 g
Phosphorus   238 mg
Potassium   305 mg
Sodium   314 mg
Protein   19g
Carbohydrates   26 g

Rice Tuna Casserole

Prep time: 5 minutes
Cook time: 35 minutes
Servings: 6

Ingredients:
½ teaspoon of basil
½ cup of chopped onion
6 ½ ounces of tuna, low sodium
1 cup of sour cream
1 sliced tomato
1 cup of cheddar cheese
1/8 teaspoon of garlic powder
3 ounces of cream cheese
3 cups of white rice, cooked

Preparations:
1. Combine together the cheddar cheese, rice and tuna in a medium bowl.
2. Grease a shallow baking dish and spoon in the mixture.

3. Beat the cream cheese until you have a smooth mixture.
4. Stir in the basil, garlic powder, onion and sour cream; spoon sour cream cheese mixture on top of tuna mixture.
5. Arrange foil over baking sheet and bake at 350 Degrees for 30 minutes.
6. Discard foil and add slices of tomato over the top. Place back to the oven and bake for 5 minutes.

Nutrition Facts per serving
Calories   348 g
Phosphorus   272 mg
Potassium   293 mg
Sodium   203 mg
Protein   17g
Carbohydrates   28 g

Cooked BBQ Shrimp

Prep time: 10 minutes
Cook time: 35 minutes
Servings: 15

Ingredients:
1 tsp of Tabasco sauce
3 tsp of cayenne pepper
2 tsp of rosemary
2 tsp of oregano
2 tsp of paprika
1 tbsp of parsley minced
1/4 cup of lemon juice
4 minced garlic cloves
2 thinly sliced lemon
1/4 cup of Worcestershire sauce
1/2 cup of chili sauce
1 cup of olive oil
2 butter sticks
7.5 lbs of shrimp, Peel, devein and wash

Preparation:
1. Combine all the ingredients without the shrimp in sauce pan.
2. Simmer on low heat for 30 minutes.

3. Meanwhile, sauté shrimp lightly in oil until partially cooked.
4. Coat the shrimp in BBQ sauce and bring to a boil.
5. Serve in bowl with enough French bread.

Nutrition Facts per serving
Calories   420 g
Phosphorus   244 mg
Potassium   423 mg
Sodium   666 mg
Protein   35 g
Carbohydrates   6 g

Extra Spicy Fried Fish
Prep time: 10 minutes
Cook time: 20 to 25 minutes
Servings: 4
Ingredients:
1 to 1 1/4 lb of catfish or any white fish filets
1/3 cup of corn meal
1/2 tsp of grated lemon zest
2 tsp of Mrs. Dash Extra Spicy Blend
1 1/2 tbsp of cumin
3 tbsp of Mrs. Dash Garlic & Herb Blend
1 tbsp of olive oil
1 1/2 tbsp of lemon juice
Preparation:
1. Heat up the oven to 400 F.
2. In a small container with lid, combine together 1 tsp Mrs. Dash Extra Spicy, 1 Tbsp Mrs. Dash Garlic & Herb, cumin, olive oil and lemon juice. Shake very well to blend.
3. Transfer the well-blended mixture to shallow plate; coat fish with the mixture on both sides.
4. Mix the remaining Mrs. Dash Seasoning Blends, corn meal and lemon rind.
5. Coat fish with the corn lemon mixture on both sides.

6. Bake until fish easily flakes with a fork, about 20 to 25 minutes. If desired, serve with extra hot pepper sauce and lemon juice.

Nutrition Facts per serving
Calories   264 g
Phosphorus   230 mg
Potassium   526 mg
Sodium   67 mg
Protein   20 g
Carbohydrates 13 g

Tuna Worcestershire Loaf

Prep time: 8 minutes
Cook time: 35 minutes
Servings: 4

Ingredients:
1/4 tsp of Worcestershire sauce
1/8 tsp of pepper
1 tbsp of onion, chopped
2 tbsp of chopped green pepper
1 cup of milk
2 eggs, beaten
12 oz of Salmon or Tuna water packed

Preparation:
1. Heat up the oven to 350 F.
2. In a large mixing bowl, mix together all the ingredients.
3. Grease loaf pan, if you don't have a loaf pan, form patties.
4. Pour into the prepared loaf pan fry the patties.
5. Bake in the oven for 35 minutes.
Serve while it's hot with Sour Creamy Dill Sauce

Nutrition Facts per serving
Calories   158 g
Phosphorus   109 mg
Potassium   141 mg
Sodium   456 mg

Protein 26 g
Carbohydrates 4 g

POULTRY AND MEAT

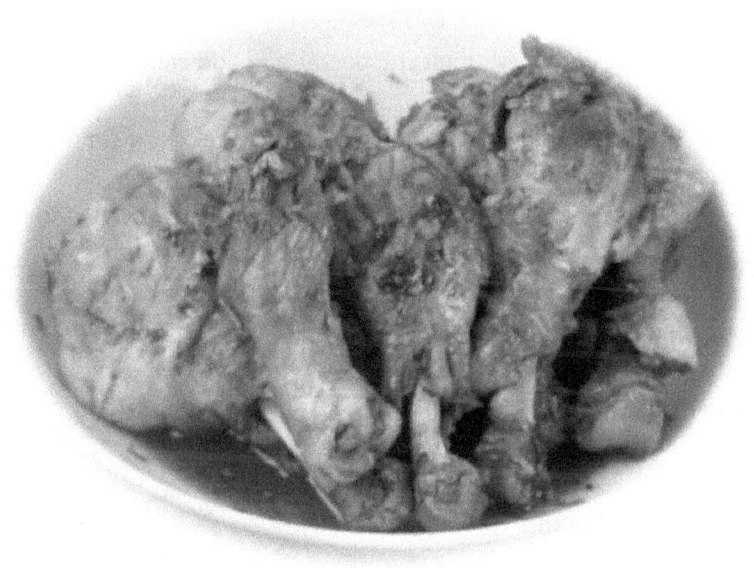

Cream Cider Chicken

Prep time: 5 minutes
Cook time: 30-35 minutes
Servings: 8

Ingredients:
1/2 cup of half and half
3/4 cup of apple cider
2 tbsp of unsalted butter
4 chicken breasts, bone-in

Preparation:
1. Over medium-high heat, melt the butter and add chicken to brown on each sides.
2. Add in the apple cider and lower to medium heat; let it simmer for 20 minutes.
3. Take the chicken out of the skillet and boil cider until the liquid is reduced to about 1/4 cup.
4. Pour in half and half and whisk until the sauce is thickened a bit.
5. Serve chicken top with the cream sauce.

Nutrition Facts per serving
Calories	186 g
Phosphorus	266 mg
Potassium	414 mg
Sodium	83 mg
Protein	27 g
Carbohydrates	1 g

Dijon Chicken Breast

Prep time: 5 minutes
Cook time: 30 minutes
Servings: 4

Ingredients:
1 tsp of curry powder
1 tsp of lemon Juice
3 tbsp of honey
1/4 cup of Dijon mustard
4 boneless chicken breasts

Preparation:
1. Heat up the oven to 350 F.
2. Arrange the chicken breast on a baking dish.
3. Mix the rest ingredients together in a bowl.
4. Brush the chicken on both side with the sauce.
5. Bake in the oven until chicken reaches an internal temperature of 165 degrees, about for 30 minutes.

Nutrition Facts per serving
Calories	189 g
Phosphorus	250 mg
Potassium	454 mg
Sodium	258 mg
Protein	25 g
Carbohydrates	14 g

Roast Chicken with Herbs

Prep time: 13 minutes
Cook time: 15 minutes per pound
Servings: 4-6

Ingredients

1 tbsp of olive oil
1 thinly sliced small lemon
2 peeled and crushed cloves garlic
2 1/2 tbsp of fresh herbs, chopped (thyme, sage etc.)
2 tbsp of unsalted butter, softened
1 whole chicken, fresh or thawed, (about 4-5 pound)

Preparation

1. Heat up the oven to 450 F.
2. Add the fresh or thawed chicken in a roasting pan.
3. In a small bowl, mix together the herbs, butter and garlic.
4. Place the herb butter mixture with the lemon slices inside the body of chicken.
5. Rub the skin all over with olive oil.
6. Roast for 15 minutes per pound in the oven, or until it reads 165 degrees in the internal temperature.
7. Drain the juices from the chicken and pour with the lemon slices over chicken.

Let it rest about 20 mins before carving.

Nutrition Facts per serving

Calories	251 g
Phosphorus	188 mg
Potassium	222 mg
Sodium	77 mg
Protein	19 g
Carbohydrates	0 g

Cheesy Basil Chicken

Prep time: 10 minutes
Cook time: 25 minutes
Servings: 4

Ingredients

(Optional) 4 fresh basil sprigs, for garnish
1/4 tsp of Mrs. Dash herb seasoning blend
1/4 tsp of garlic powder
1 tbsp of grated parmesan cheese
1/4 cup of fresh basil
1/3 cup of trans-fat free margarine
4 skinless chicken breasts, halved

Preparation

1. Heat up the oven to 325° Degrees.
2. In a glass baking pan, arrange each chicken halves and use a fork to Pierce several
holes into each chicken to allow chicken absorb mixture season as it cooks.
3. Heat margarine in the microwave in a glass mixing bowl. Begin at 15 seconds and stirring to distribute heat.
4. Add garlic powder, basil, Mrs. Dash and parmesan cheese to melted margarine. Whisk mixture using a fork.
5. Pour sauce on top of chicken breasts evenly, make sure the cheese is evenly distributed.
6. Baked in the oven uncovered, baste chicken with sauce in the pan every 10 minutes as you cook, about 25 minutes or until no more pink and the juices runs clear.

Nutrition Facts per serving
Calories   252 g
Phosphorus   210 mg
Potassium   246 mg
Sodium   231 mg
Protein   27 g
Carbohydrates   0 g

Turkey Sliders with Aioli Mixture

Prep time: 12minutes
Cook time: 15 minutes
Servings: 3

Ingredients

For the Aioli:

1 tsp of chopped tarragon
2 tbsp of mayonnaise
2 tbsp of peaches, pureed

For the Turkey Sliders:

1 tsp of poultry seasoning
1/2 cup of arugula
1/4 cup of diced red onion
1/3 cup of chopped parsley
6 slider buns
450 g of ground turkey
1 tsp of garlic powder
1/2 tbsp of dijon mustard

Preparations

1. Warm up your BBQ grill for high-medium heat. Combine together the turkey, red onion, parsley, garlic powder, poultry season and dijon in a mixing bowl and shape into six patties.
2. Cook turkey sliders for 5 to 6 mins on each side or until it reads 165F when an instant read thermometer is inserted into the center.
3. Spread aioli mixture over the base and top of the slider buns. Arrange 1 patty over one bottom bun then top with arugula and place top bun.

Nutrition Facts per serving
Calories	257 g
Phosphorus	240 mg
Potassium	330 mg
Sodium	257 mg
Protein	16g
Carbohydrates	33 g

Grilled Garlic Lemon Chicken Kebabs

Prep time: 3 hours
Cook time: 20 minutes
Servings: 4-6

Ingredients

1 tsp of white wine vinegar
2 bay leaves, cut in half
1 tbsp of chopped fresh herbs (thyme, sage etc.)
1 peeled and crushed clove garlic
3 tbsp of olive oil
2 lemons
4 skinless, boneless chicken thighs

Preparation

1. Chop the chicken thighs into thick piece and add in a bowl.
2. Grate one tsp of lemon zest and juice the rest lemon.
3. Combine oil, vinegar, herbs and garlic in a bowl, add the chicken and cover and marinate about 3 hours, or overnight.
4. Cut the second lemon into thick 4 slices, then slice each of the slices into another 4 pieces.
5. Pierce each lemon slices and chicken pieces on a wooden skewer alternatively, making it firm as possible then add lemon piece lastly. Do the same for each skewer.
6. Grill about 10 minutes each side, (any grilling style you choose) until done.

Nutrition Facts per serving
Calories   362 g
Phosphorus   238 mg
Potassium   404 mg
Sodium   119 mg
Protein   27 g
Carbohydrates   6 g

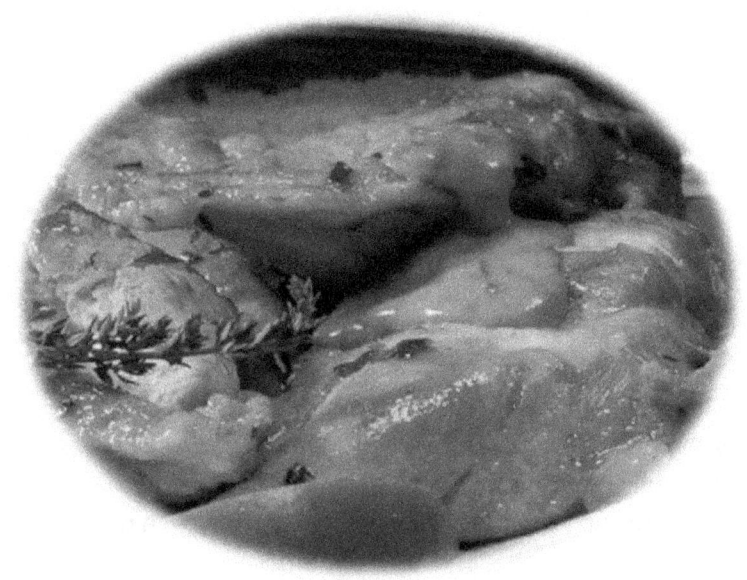

Broccoli Turkey Casserole

Prep time: 15minutes
Cook time: 25-30 minutes
Servings: 8

Ingredients

3 cups of broccoli florets
4 cups of cooked turkey, cut into 3/4-inch pieces
1 cup of chopped pepper (red, green or yellow)
2 tsp of curry powder
3 cups of white bread, diced medium
Ground pepper
2 minced garlic cloves
2 cups of chicken broth, no salt added
1 cup of 2% milk
1/4 cup of olive oil or canola plus 2 tablespoons
1 small finely diced yellow onion
1/4 cup of all-purpose flour

Preparations

1. Warm up the oven to 400 Degrees.

2. Heat quarter cup of olive or canola oil over medium heat in a medium pot.
3. Add garlic and onion; cook about 7 minutes until onion is soft a bit but not browned.
4. Whisk in flour continuously for one minute. Fold in chicken broth and milk, whisking rapidly until you have a smooth mixture.
5. Cook and stir every now and then until it comes to a simmer. Add curry powder and season with pepper, stir. Add sweet pepper and broccoli, keep cooking, about 5 minutes until it starts to soften.
6. Add the turkey and stir everything together.
7. Pour the turkey mixture into 8-inches square baking dish.
8. Toss bread with the reserve two tbsp of oil in a small bowl until coated.
9. Add the bread on top the turkey and bake in the oven until bread is golden brown and sauce is bubbling, about 15 minutes

Nutrition Facts per serving
Calories   380 g
Phosphorus   227 mg
Potassium   472 mg
Sodium   113 mg
Protein   26 g
Carbohydrates   23 g

Starter Chicken Tacos
Prep time: 10 minutes
Cook time: 20 minutes
Ingredients
Servings: 4
2 sliced green onions (scallions)
1/4 cup of sour cream
1 cup of shredded or chopped iceberg lettuce
8 corn tortillas
1 juice of lime
1 1/2 tsp of salt-free taco seasoning
1 lbs of skinless, boneless chicken breasts
1/2 cup of chopped cilantro
Preparation

1. Boil chicken in a skillet over medium high heat for 20 minutes.
2. When it done, take out the chicken and shred into bite-size pieces.
3. Toss chicken with lime juice and seasoning.
4. Stuff each tortillas with lettuce and shredded chicken.
5. Top with cilantro, green onions, sour cream or other garnishes.

Nutrition Facts per serving
Calories   141 g
Phosphorus   155 mg
Potassium   220 mg
Sodium   50 mg
Protein   14 g
Carbohydrates   9 g

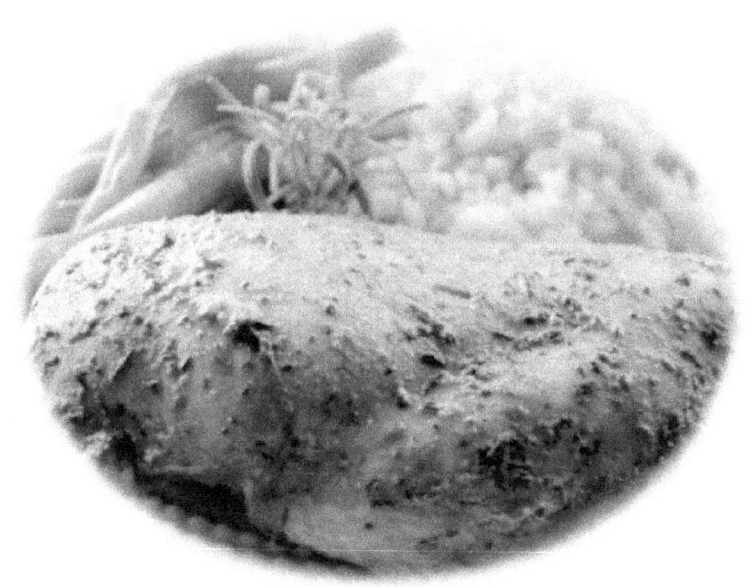

Herb Coated Bread Chicken

Serving: 4

Cook time: varies

Ingredients

1 lbs of boneless or 1 1/2 lbs "bone in" chicken breasts

1 1/2 slices whole wheat bread

1/4 tsp of fresh ground black pepper

1/4 tsp of paprika

1/4 tsp of tarragon

1/4 tsp of oregano

1/4 tsp of thyme

1/4 tsp of basil

Preparation

1. Heat up the oven to 400 F.

1. Combine spices, herbs with the bread in a food processor or blender. Mix well.

2. Place the chicken in a bowl, add cold water and rinse. Dip chicken in bread/herb mixture.

3. Bake chicken in the oven in a single layer (if boneless, for 20 minutes, if bone in, bake for 50 minutes).

Nutrition Facts per serving

Calories	172 g
Phosphorus	249 mg
Potassium	444 mg
Sodium	180 mg
Protein	27 g
Carbohydrates	7 g

Honey Vinegar Molasses Pork

Prep time: 10 minutes
Cook time: 25-30 minutes
Servings: 6

Ingredients

1/4 cup of cold water
1 tbsp of cornstarch
1 1/3 lbs of pork, about 3/4 inch thick
1 tbsp of canola oil
2 tbsp of molasses
2 tbsp of dijon mustard
1/4 cup of balsamic vinegar
1/4 cup of honey
1/4 cup of water
2 tbsp of brown sugar

Preparation

1. Add sugar, water, honey, vinegar, dijon mustard and molasses in a small bowl and stir until finely blended.
2. Slice the pork into 2 inch long by 1/4 inch pieces.
3. Brown pork for 2 minutes on each side in a large fry pan with oil over medium heat.
4. Add in the sauce, lower the heat to medium-low, simmer covered for 15 minutes.
5. Dissolve cornstarch in cold water and pour over the pork.
6. Turn heat up to medium and heat until it boils, stirring frequently.
7. Simmer on medium heat without covering until sauce thickens, about 5 minutes.

Nutrition Facts per serving

Calories	241 g
Phosphorus	170 mg
Potassium	392 mg
Sodium	165 mg
Protein	21 g
Carbohydrates	22 g

SOUP AND STEW

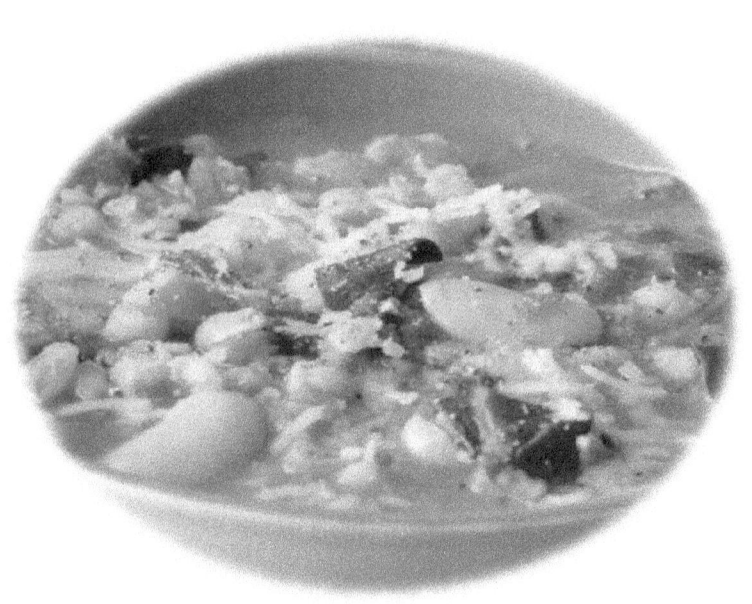

Corn Celery and Fennel Soup

Prep time: 12 minutes
Cook time: 30-35 minutes
Servings: 12

Ingredients

2 liters of cold water
Tarragon to taste
Black pepper to taste
2 cups of chopped fennel
6 cloves garlic
1 chopped celery stalk
2 chopped onions or leeks
2 pounds of frozen corn
2 tablespoon of vegetable oil
Shrimp shells

Preparations

1. Add oil in a sauce pan and sauté shrimp shells until color turns pink.
2. Add onion, garlic, corn, celery and fennel and sauté until onions are tender and translucent and flavored.
3. Add in water and bring to a boil. Simmer for about 30 minutes.
4. Transfer soup to a blender (be careful of the hot liquid) and blend.
5. Strain soup to remove any excess fibers.
6. Adjust seasonings with tarragon and ground black pepper.

Nutrition Facts per serving
Calories   112 g
Phosphorus   76 mg
Potassium   298 mg
Sodium   16 mg
Protein   3 g
Carbohydrates   22 g

Sea Coast Roasted Red Pepper Soup

Prep time: 15 minutes
Cook time: 35 minutes
Servings: 6

Ingredients

1/4 cup of toasted cashews or almonds
1 tbsp of red wine vinegar
2/3 cup of nonfat dry milk
2 cups chicken broth (low sodium) or water
1 (28 ounce) can of diced tomatoes
3 fresh roasted red peppers
1/2 cup of lentils, rinsed and sorted
1 tsp of paprika
6 diced garlic cloves
2 large diced onions
2 tbsp of olive oil

Preparation

1. Sauté onions in olive oil, stirring not too often until onions are tender and caramelized.
2. Add paprika and garlic and cook for 2 minutes and then add tomatoes, lentils, 1 cup broth and peppers. Bring to boil, simmer on low heat, cover with the lid and cook about 30 min or until lentils are soft.
3. Whirl soup in a food processor or blender in batches, until smooth.
4. Add vinegar and dry milk to the final batch. Stir well.
5. If desired, season with extra vinegar to taste and if the soup is too thick, add a more broth to desired consistency
6. To serve, garnish with a sparkle of toasted cashews or almonds and a drizzle of oil.

Nutrition Facts per serving

Calories	112 g
Phosphorus	83 mg
Potassium	370 mg
Sodium	128 mg
Protein	11 g
Carbohydrates	31 g

Low Sodium White Sauce

Prep time: 3 minutes
Cook time: 4 minutes
Servings: 4

Ingredients

1/2 tsp of fresh parsley, basil, or other herbs or 1 tsp of dried
1/4 tsp of dry mustard
1 cup of heavy cream
2 tbsp of unsalted butter or margarine
1/4 tsp of paprika
2 tbsp of flour

Preparation

1. Mix butter or margarine with flour in a small microwave-safe bowl.
2. Place in the microwave for half a minute, stir and microwave another half minute.
3. Add spices and cream, stir and microwave for 60 seconds, stir again. Microwave for 1 minute. If sauce is not thick enough, add 1 minute more.

Nutrition Facts per serving

Calories	273 g
Phosphorus	43 mg
Potassium	54 mg
Sodium	25 mg
Protein	2 g
Carbohydrates	5 g

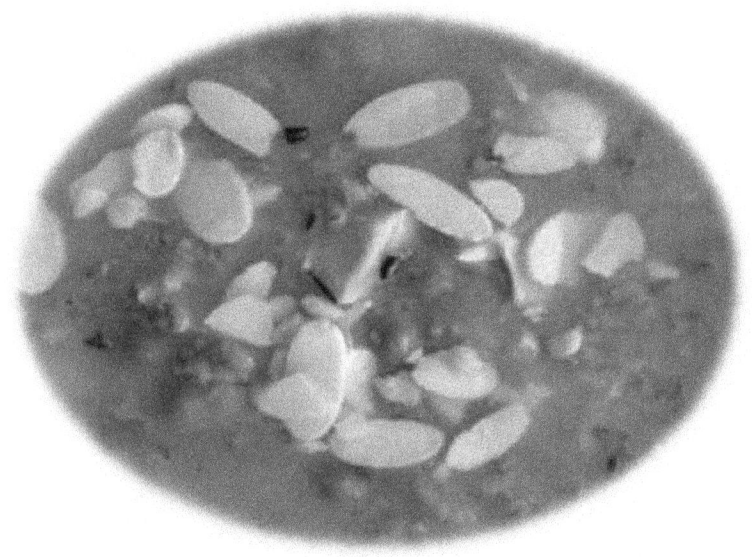

Chicken With Mushrooms Soup

Prep time: 15 minutes
Cook time: 20-25 minutes
Servings: 6

Ingredients

2 tbsp of lime juice
1/2 sliced yellow onion
1 sliced red bell pepper
10 white button mushrooms, quartered
1 can of lite coconut milk
1 inch sliced ginger
1 chopped lemon grass stalk
1 tsp of chili sauce or chili flakes
1 tbsp of brown or white sugar
1/2 tbsp of fish sauce
4 cups of low sodium broth or Simple Chicken Broth
1 lbs of chicken breast or shrimp, cut into bite size pieces

Preparation

1. Spray a nonstick cooking spray on a large pot, add shrimp or chicken and cook over medium heat until evenly browned.

2. Add ginger, lemongrass, chili sauce, sugar, fish sauce, and broth. Bring to a boil.
3. Reduce to low-medium heat and simmer about 10 to 15 minutes.
4. Add onion, bell pepper, mushrooms and coconut milk and simmer for 5 more minutes.
5. Mix in lime juice just before serving.

Nutrition Facts per serving
Calories	233 g
Phosphorus	382 mg
Potassium	800 mg
Sodium	300 mg
Protein	32 g
Carbohydrates	9 g

Beef Veggie Barley Soup

Prep Time: 15 minutes
Cook Time: 1 hour 43 minutes
Servings: 10

Ingredients

1/4 tsp of dried thyme
1/2 cup of barley
3 cups of water
1 (16 ounces) package of vegetables, frozen
1/4 cup of vegetable oil, divided
1/2 cup of sliced mushrooms
1 (14.5 ounces) can of chicken broth, low sodium
1/2 tsp of minced garlic
2 diced carrots
2 potatoes, soaked and diced
1 cup of onion, chopped
2 pounds of beef stew meat, diced into 1 inch cubes
1/2 tsp of black pepper

Preparation

1. Season the beef stew meat using black pepper.
2. Arrange the season beef onto the skillet, and add 2 tbsp of oil to stew pot. Sauté for 5 minutes, add two extra tbsp of oil, add onions, mushrooms and carrots.
3. Sauté for 5 additional minutes, stirring regularly. Pour in thyme and garlic and sauté for three minutes.
4. Add cups of water and broth into the skillet, then add barley, potatoes and mixed vegetables. Stir and keep cooking until heated through. Cover with the lid and simmer on low heat for 1 to 1 1/2 hours

Nutrition Facts per serving
Calories   270 g
Phosphorus   250 mg
Potassium   678 mg
Sodium   105 mg
Protein   23 g
Carbohydrates   22 g

Fancy Chili

Prep time: 5 minutes
Cook time: 1 hour 5 minutes
Servings: 6

Ingredients

1/4 tsp of Cajun seasoning
1 tsp of dried basil
1/2 tsp of dried thyme
1/2 tsp of dried oregano
1/4 tsp of ground cumin
1 tbsp of garlic powder
2 tbsp of chili powder
1 chopped orange or red bell pepper
1 (4 oz) can of green chili pepper, chopped
2 cups of water
1, 8 oz can of tomato sauce (look for unsalted)
1 large onion
1 lbs of lean ground beef

Preparation

1. Cook beef in a large pot, over medium high heat until browned.
2. Add onion, stir and cook until onion is soft.
3. Stir in bell pepper, 2 cups water, tomato sauce, spices and green chilies.
4. Heat until it boils then reduce to medium-low heat and simmer for about one hour.

Nutrition Facts per serving
Calories   225 g
Phosphorus   168 mg
Potassium   490 mg
Sodium   218 mg
Protein   21 g
Carbohydrates 10 g

Piecrust Chicken Stew

Prep time: 45 minutes
Cook time: 60 minutes
Servings: 8

Ingredients

1 frozen piecrust, cooked and broken into bite-size pieces
1/2 cup of light cream
1/2 cup of fresh frozen sweet peas, thawed
2 tbsp of chicken bouillon powder (salt-free)
1 tbsp of Italian seasoning (salt-free)
1 tbsp of black pepper
1/4 cup of diced celery
1/2 cup diced onion
1/2 cup of fresh carrots, diced
1/2 cup of flour
1/4 cup of canola oil
2 quarts of chicken stock, low-sodium
1 1/2 pounds of natural fresh skinless, boneless, chicken breast

Preparations

1. Pound the chicken to make it tenderer, Place in the freezer for 30 minutes, (this will allow you cut easily), then cube.
2. In large stockpot, place the stock and chicken, cook for 30 minutes on medium-high heat.
3 While the chicken is cooking, mix flour with oil until finely blended. Then slowly stir the flour mixture into chicken mixture until slightly thickened. Reduce to low or medium-low heat and cook for 15 minutes.
4. Add bouillon, Italian seasoning, celery, onion, carrots and black pepper. Cook for 15 extra minutes. Remove from heat, and then add cream and peas. Stir together until well mixed.
5. Pour into mugs and serve garnish with equal amounts of piecrust on top.

Nutrition Facts per serving
Calories   419 g
Phosphorus   229 mg
Potassium   412 mg
Sodium   296 mg

Protein   30 g
Carbohydrates   24 g

Seasoned Chicken and Gnocchi

Prep time: 15 minutes
Cook time: 30- 45 minutes
Servings: 6

Ingredients

¼ cup of chopped fresh parsley
½ cup of finely diced fresh carrots
½ cup of finely diced fresh onions
½ cup of finely diced fresh celery
6 cups of reduced-sodium chicken stock
1 tbsp of low sodium better than Bouillon Chicken Base
¼ cup of grape seed or light olive oil
1 lbs of store bought gnocchi
2 lbs of chicken breast
1 tsp of Italian seasoning
1 tsp of black pepper

Preparations

1. Add oil to a deep saucepan over high heat.
2. Add chicken and cook until golden brown on all sides.
3. Add onions, carrots and celery and keep cooking until union translucent.
4. Pour in the chicken stock and cook about 20–30 minutes.
5. Reduce to medium heat, stir in Italian seasoning, chicken bouillon and black pepper. 6. Pour in the gnocchi, cook for additional 15 minutes, stirring frequently.

Turn heat off and garnish with parsley to serve.

Nutrition Facts per serving
Calories   362 g
Phosphorus   295 mg
Potassium   485 mg
Sodium   121 mg
Protein   28 g
Carbohydrates   38 g

Creamy Potato Soup

Servings: 6

Ingredients

1/2 cup of sour cream, fat free
4 cups of skim milk
4 oz of shredded Monterey jack cheese, reduce fat
2 large potatoes
1/2 tsp of pepper
1/3 cup of flour

Preparation

1. Arrange the potatoes in the oven and bake at 400 degrees until potatoes are tender.
2. Once the potatoes are cool enough to handle, cut in half lengthwise and scoop the pulp out.
3. In a large stockpot, add flour and gently stir in milk, until well blended.
4. Add pepper and the scooped potato pulp.
5. Cook and stir regularly over medium heat until bubbly and thick.
6. Stir in the cheese, until it's melted. Turn heat off and stir in sour cream.

Nutrition Facts per serving

Calories	216 g
Phosphorus	326 mg
Potassium	594 mg
Sodium	272 mg
Protein	15 g
Carbohydrates	29 g

Rice And Chicken Carrot Soup

Prep time: 10 minutes
Cook time: 25 minutes
Servings: 8

Ingredients

2 tablespoon of lime juice
2 skinless, boneless chicken breasts, cooked and cut into cube sizes
10 cups chicken/vegetable broth (No salt added)
1 bay leaf
4 fresh thyme sprigs
½ teaspoon of fresh ground black pepper
¾ Cup of instant white rice, uncooked
2 tablespoon of extra virgin oil
1 Cup of chopped baby carrot
1 Cup of diced celery
1 Cup of finely chopped white onion

Preparations

1. Sautee onion, celery and carrot in oil in a large skillet until softened.
2. Add rice, fresh thyme, bay leaf, pepper and stock. Bring to a boil
3. Reduce to low heat, and let it simmer for 15 minutes.
4. Add chicken cubes and cook on low heat for 10 minutes.
5. Discard the bay leaf and add in the lime juice.

Nutrition Facts per serving
Calories	160 g
Phosphorus	90 mg
Potassium	251 mg
Sodium	221 mg
Protein	14 g
Carbohydrates	19 g

SALAD RECIPES

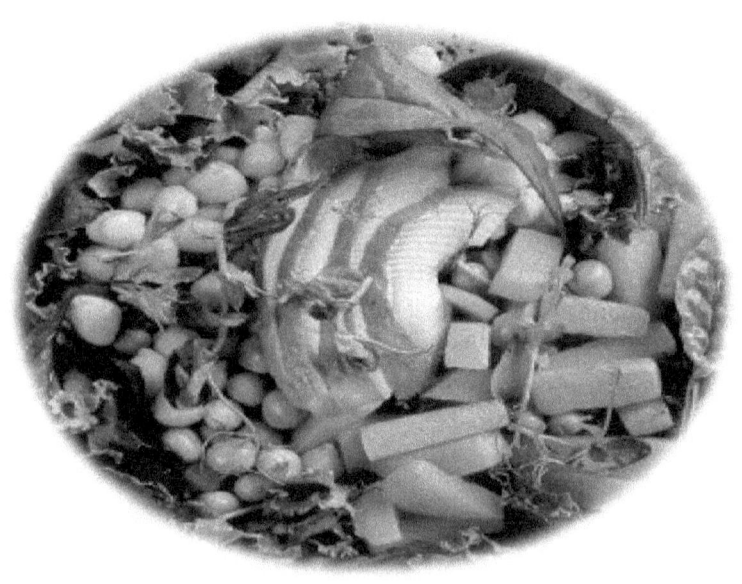

Low Protein Strawberry Salad

Prep time: 15 minutes

Servings: 6

Ingredients

Dressing:

1 teaspoon of soy sauce (low sodium)

1 teaspoon of curry powder

2 tablespoon of brown sugar

1 minced garlic clove

1/3 cup of white wine vinegar

1/2 cup of vegetable oil

Salad:

2 cups of mandarin orange segments

1/2 cup of unsalted pretzels, crushed

2 cups of strawberries, sliced

1 cup of green or red grapes, halved

1/2 cup of toasted slivered almonds

10 cups of torn salad greens

Preparations

1. Toss the strawberries and salad greens together in a bowl
2. Add all the dressing ingredients in a container, cover and shake well.
3. Toss the salad with dressing and sprinkle with pretzels and almonds. Serve.

Nutrition Facts per serving

Calories	256 g
Phosphorus	85.9 mg
Potassium	344 mg
Sodium	41 mg
Protein	4 g
Carbohydrates	24 g

Rice Vinegar Cucumber Salad

Prep time: 70 minutes

Servings: 10

Ingredients

2 tablespoon of toasted white sesame seeds, for garnish

1/3 cup of sugar

½ cup of water

½ cup of rice vinegar

1 diced red onion

3 English peeled cucumbers and slice thinly into rounds

Preparations

1. Add the cucumber rounds and red onion into a bowl.
2. Stir sugar, rice vinegar and water together and pour over onion and cucumber.
3. Cover tightly and marinate for 60 minutes.
4. Transfer into a Plate and top with sesame seeds to garnish.

Nutrition Facts per serving

Calories	51 g
Phosphorus	29 mg
Potassium	130 mg
Sodium	5 mg
Protein	1 g
Carbohydrates	24 g

Creamy Pickles Pasta Salad

Servings: 8

Ingredients

1/8 tsp of ground mustard
1/4 cup of Refrigerator chopped Pickles
1 chopped stalk celery
2 tbsp of grated carrot
1 tsp of onion powder
8 oz medium shells pasta
1/2 cup of mayonnaise
1/2 cup of sour cream
1/2 tsp of celery seed

Preparation

1. Cook pasta the way instructed in the package directions, rinse cooked pasta with cold water and set aside.
2. Whisk sour cream, mayonnaise, ground mustard, onion powder and celery seed in a different bowl.
3. Stir the mixture into cooked pasta and mix in the chopped pickles.
4. Garnish with carrot and celery.

Nutrition Facts per serving

Calories	188 g
Phosphorus	56 mg
Potassium	90 mg
Sodium	134 mg
Protein	4 g
Carbohydrates	23 g

Roasted Peanuts Salad with Chili-Lime Sauce

Servings: 4-6

Ingredients

1/2 cup of roasted, (whole or chopped) unsalted peanuts
1/2 cup of shredded carrot
1/2 head of shredded red cabbage
1 bunch of cilantro
1 chopped red onion
2 cups of sweet corn kernels
2-3 tbsp of Thai sweet chili sauce
2-3 minced garlic cloves
2 lime juice and zest

Preparation

1. Mix garlic, sweet chili sauce and lime zest and juice in a small bowl.
2. In a separate large bowl, Combine the vegetables ingredients, drizzle dressing over the salad and gently toss. Serve immediately or chill before serving.

Nutrition Facts per serving

Calories	115 g
Phosphorus	68 mg
Potassium	225 mg
Sodium	120 mg
Protein	3 g
Carbohydrates	21 g

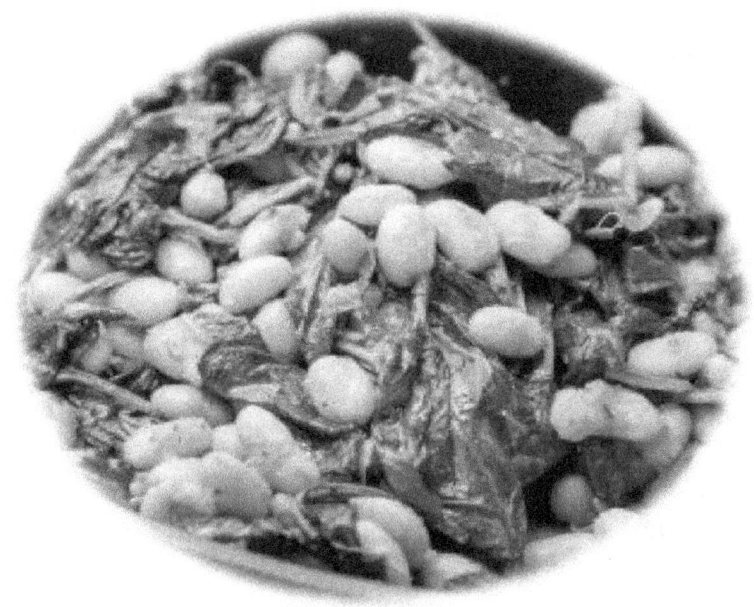

Persimmon Pomegranate Salad
Servings: 12
Ingredients
8 oz of goat cheese, crumbled
2-3 fresh persimmons
2 tbsp of olive oil
1/4 cup of raspberry vinegar
2 tbsp of fresh basil leaves or 1/4 tsp of dried
1/2 cup of chopped pecans or cashews
1/2 cup of pomegranate seeds
6 cups of baby spinach or mixed salad greens
Preparation
1. Wash greens well to remove all dirt, drain well.
2. Toss greens with the rest ingredients and place crumbled goat cheese over the salad. Chill and serve.

Nutrition Facts per serving
Calories	134 g
Phosphorus	68 mg
Potassium	86 mg
Sodium	105 mg
Protein	5 g

Carbohydrates   9 g

Green molasses Salad

Servings: 4

Ingredients

(Optional) 1/4 cup of nuts
1 pinch of allspice
1 tsp of mustard
1/2 cup of olive oil
1/4 cup of fresh parsley
2 tbsp of lemon juice
1/4 cup of pomegranate molasses
1/4 cup of Greek or plain yogurt
1 ounces of chive flowers, edible flowers or violets
3 ounces of goat cheese
1 diced pear
1 cup of frozen peas or sugar snap peas, Cut in pods into thirds
1 cucumber, Chop into disk then quarter
4 cups of spring greens, tear into bite size pieces

Preparation

1. Combine the greens, cucumber, pear and snap peas in a bowl. (If snap peas is frozen, thaw at room temperature for 30 minutes)
2. Mix the chive flowers with goat cheese, then cut into half inch pieces.
3. Blend allspice, mustard, olive oil, parsley, lemon juice, molasses and yogurt in a food processor or blender.
4. Pour the dressing over salad in a bowl. Toss to coat.
5. Sprinkle the salad with nuts (optional), goat cheese and flowers.

Nutrition Facts per serving
Calories   212 g
Phosphorus   164 mg
Potassium   218 mg
Sodium   127 mg
Protein   11 g
Carbohydrates 11 g

Toasted Almond Summer Salad

Servings: 4

Ingredients

1/8 tsp of pepper
1 tsp of sugar
2 tbsp of balsamic vinegar
1/4 cup of olive oil
1/4 cup of shredded parmesan cheese
1/4 cup of slivered almonds, toasted
1 small purple onion, sliced in rings
1 (11 ounce) can of chilled mandarin oranges, drained
6-8 sliced strawberries
1 small of head butter lettuce, torn

Preparation

1. In a large salad bowl, combine together the salad ingredients.
2. Get a jar and combine pepper, sugar, balsamic vinegar and olive oil.
3. Cover the jar and shake until well mixed.
4. Pour dressing over the salad, gently toss to coat. Serve immediately.

Nutrition Facts per serving

Calories	250 g
Phosphorus	104 mg
Potassium	265 mg
Sodium	95 mg
Protein	5 g
Carbohydrates	14 g

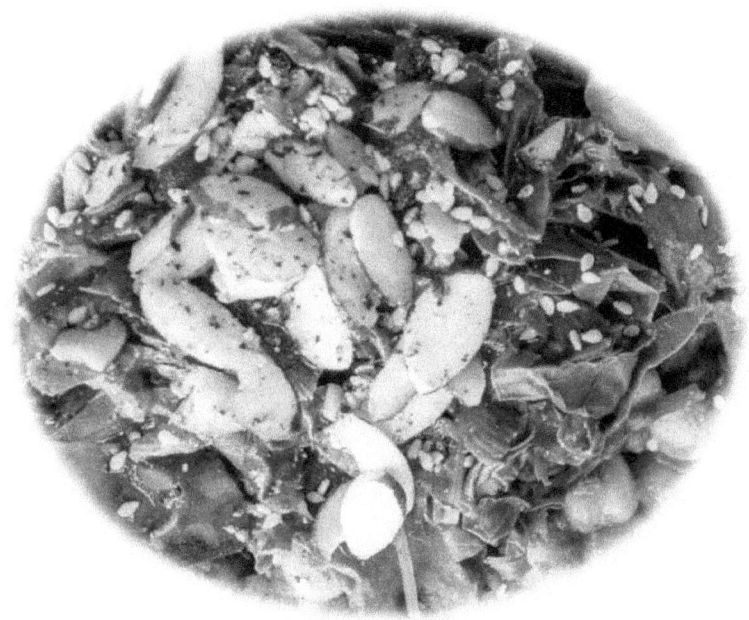

Lemon tarragon Orzo Salad

Cook time: 8 to 10 minutes
Servings: 4

Ingredients

1 tablespoon of extra virgin olive oil
2 tablespoon of lemon juice
2 tablespoon of chopped parsley
2 tablespoon of chopped tarragon
1 diced green onion
1 diced red pepper
1 cup of orzo pasta or any desired small shapes pasta
1/2 teaspoon of black pepper
1 teaspoon of garlic, minced

Preparations

1. Cook orzo for 8 to 10 minutes in boiling water and if any other pasta, cook according to packet instructions. Drain and place under running water to cool. Toss with the rest ingredients and serve.

Nutrition Facts per serving
Calories   148 g
Phosphorus   65 mg
Potassium   164 mg
Sodium   6 mg
Protein   4 g
Carbohydrates   24 g

Pear And wine vinegar Arugula Salad

Servings: 6

Ingredients

1 minced shallot
1 sliced pear
6 cups of arugula (Rinse and trimmed stems off)
3 tablespoon of red wine vinegar
Cracked black pepper
1 teaspoon of Dijon mustard
2/3 cup of extra virgin olive oil

Preparations

1. Combine Dijon mustard, black pepper, red wine vinegar and shallot in blender. Fold in the olive oil to emulsify.
2. Combine together arugula and pear and toss to coat with the dressing.

Nutrition Facts per serving
Calories   250 g
Phosphorus   18 mg
Potassium   172 mg
Sodium   19 mg
Protein   0.8 g
Carbohydrates   6 g

Asian Apple With sesame seeds Slaw

Servings: 4

Ingredients

2 tablespoon of Splenda or sugar
1/4 cup of rice wine vinegar
1/4 cup of lime juice
1 teaspoon of sesame oil
1/2 cup of vegetable oil
2 tablespoon of toasted sesame seeds
1/2 cup of cilantro
1/2 cup of chopped celery
1 shredded granny smith apple
3 green onions, chopped
1/2 cup of chopped red pepper
4 cups of finely shredded cabbage

Preparations

1. In a large mixing bowl, combine together all vegetables, fruit and fresh herbs.
2. Whisk vinegar, lime juice, oils and sugar together in a separate bowl.
3. Pour salad dressing over the slaw, toss and top with toasted sesame seeds to garnish.

Nutrition Facts per serving

Calories	186 g
Phosphorus	25 mg
Potassium	164 mg
Sodium	17 mg
Protein	1 g
Carbohydrates	10 g

VEGETARIAN AND VEGETABLES

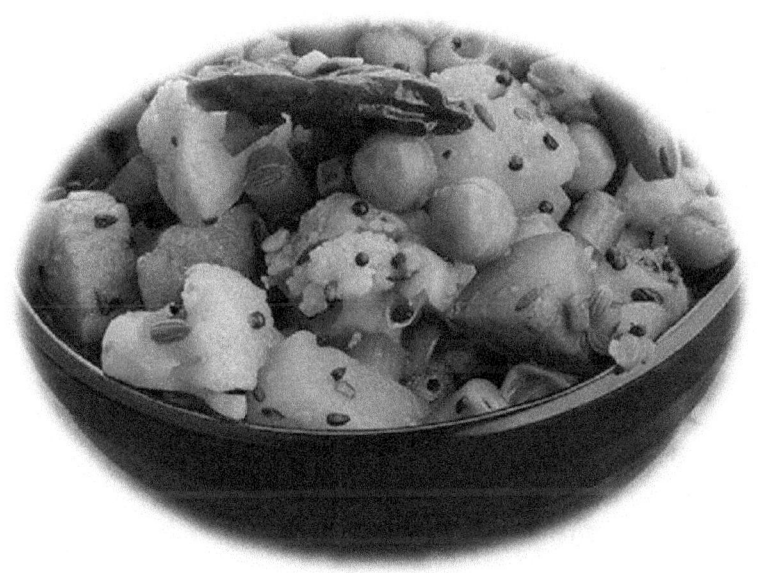

Roasted Brussels sprouts

Prep time: 5 minutes
Cook time: 10 minutes
Servings: 4-6

Ingredients

1/4 cup of fruit or herb flavored vinegar
2-4 tbsp of fresh grated Parmesan Cheese
1-2 tbsp of olive oil
2 cups of Brussels sprouts

Preparation

1. Heat up the oven to 450 F.
2. Rinse off old Brussels sprouts leaves in cold water to remove dirt. Leave the smaller sprouts whole and slice the larger sprouts in half.
3. Add olive oil to sprouts and toss to coat.
4. Place on a lightly greased baking sheet.
5. Roast until sprouts are fork tender, about 10 minutes.
6. Sprinkle roasted sprouts with the Parmesan cheese and fruit vinegar

Nutrition Facts per serving

Calories	68 g
Phosphorus	59 mg
Potassium	182 mg
Sodium	70 mg
Protein	3 g
Carbohydrates	4 g

Homemade Herb Rolls

Prep time: 1 hour 20 minutes
Cook time: 20-25 minutes
Servings: 18

Ingredients

1 large egg, beaten
1/2 cup of milk
4 tbsp of mixed rosemary, chives, thyme, parsley
2 tbsp of olive oil
3 1/2 cups of flour
3 tbsp of sugar
1 package of dry yeast

Preparation

1. Pour 1/4 cup of lukewarm water in a bowl, sprinkle yeast into the water. Allow to stand 5 minutes, and then add sugar.
2. Pour the flour into a large bowl, make a well and add milk, olive oil, herbs and beaten egg but reserve 1 tbsp for brushing. Mix well.
3. Knead dough for about 10 minutes on floured surface/board until it's smooth and elastic and form balls. (Half ounce each and about 1 1/2" across)
4. Grease a cookie sheet and Place the rolls. Allow to rise about an hour to twice the original side.
5. Heat up the oven to 350 F.
6. Use the reserved egg to brush the rolls all over.
7. Bake in the oven until golden browned, about 20-25 minutes.

Nutrition Facts per serving
Calories   117 g
Phosphorus   43 mg
Potassium   75 mg
Sodium   8 mg
Protein   3 g
Carbohydrates 21 g

Lemon Cream Chess Pie

Prep time: 10 minutes
Cook time: 45-55 minutes
Servings: 8

Ingredients

Fresh mint sprigs to garnish
1 cup of whipped cream
1/3 cup of fresh lemon juice
4 large eggs
2 tbsp of lemon zest
3 tbsp of cornstarch
6 tbsp of unsalted butter, (3/4 stick)
1 1/2 cups of sugar
1 9" single pie crust

Preparation

1. Warm up the oven to 350 F.
2. Bake the pie crust per package instructions or about 8 minutes until golden brown.
Let cool.
2. In a large bowl, beat together the butter and sugar until fluffy.
3. Add the lemon zest and cornstarch. Beat in the eggs, one by one and then beat in the juice of the lemon.
4. Pour mixture into the pie shell.
5. Bake in the oven, about 40-45 minutes, until the top is golden and filling is set. Let cool. Serve with small sprig of mint and a little amount of whipped cream.

Nutrition Facts per serving
Calories   443 g
Phosphorus   63 mg
Potassium   73 mg
Sodium   161 mg
Protein   6 g
Carbohydrates   59 g

Macaroni & Cheese In A Flash

Prep time: 5 minutes
Cook time: 5-7 minutes
Servings: 4

Ingredients

1/4 tsp of dry ground mustard
1 tsp of unsalted butter
1/2 cup of grated cheddar cheese
3 cups of water
1 cup of noodles, uncooked (any shape)

Preparation

1. Cook noodles until they are tender, about 5-7 minutes. Drain.
2. While noodles are still really hot, sprinkle with grated cheddar cheese then stir in ground mustard and butter.

Nutrition Facts per serving
Calories   152 g
Phosphorus   107 mg
Potassium   52 mg
Sodium   90 mg
Protein   7 g
Carbohydrates   18 g

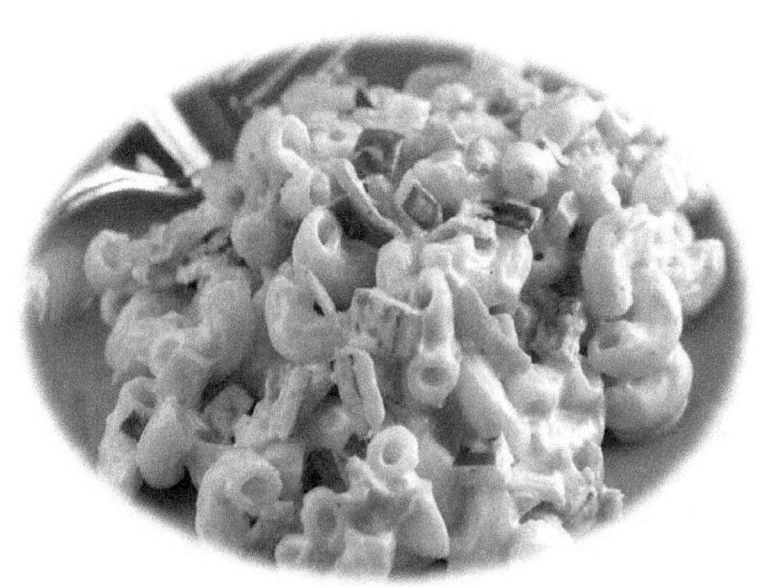

Blasted Cheese Garnished Vegetables

Prep time: 15 minutes

Cook time: 37 minutes

Servings: 6

Ingredients

Parmesan cheese to taste

1/4 cup of fruit vinegar

2 tbsp of olive oil

1 beet

1 sliced yam

1 diced onion

3/4 cup of diced carrots

1 Yukon gold potato, cut in cubes

Preparation

1. Slice the vegetables lengthwise or coin shaped into equal sized pieces.
2. Heat oil in the oven in a flat metal pan at 500 degree, for 2 minutes.
3. Add onion, carrots, and potatoes, about 10 minutes.
4. Cook stirring, for extra 5 minutes, add beets and yam, cook for 20 minutes, stirring twice at equal intervals. 10 minutes.
5. Remove and, sprinkle with grated parmesan and vinegar and serve.

Nutrition Facts per serving

Calories	247 g
Phosphorus	67 mg
Potassium	243 mg
Sodium	62 mg
Protein	5 g
Carbohydrates	40 g

Pinto Beans And Parslied Onions

Servings: 8-12

Ingredients

4 cups of low sodium pinto beans
1/2 tsp of curry powder
6 cups of sliced onions
1 tbsp of oil
2 tbsp of butter
2 cups of low salt chicken broth
1 large lemon
1/2 cup of fresh dill, wash and dry
1 cup of curly parsley
1 cup of Italian parsley, flat-leafed, wash and dry
Pepper to taste

Preparation

1. Cut off any thick stems from parsley and dill and slice into 1/2 – 1 inch size pieces; set aside.
2. Cut the lemon into half and squeeze out the juice; set aside.
3. Add the chicken broth and halved lemon in a small saucepan. Cook until it starts to boil, reduce heat, cover and simmer.
4. Heat the oil and butter in a large saucepan, add onions and cook until it's wilted and golden.
5. Stir in the parsley, dill and curry powder. Add the lemon halves and broth.
6. Slowly Cook without covering until parsley is tender and the broth has reduced.
(This helps the parsley to retain its brilliant color.)
7. Add in the beans, stir and add the juice of lemon, cook until heated through.
Discard the lemon halves. Add pepper to taste.

Nutrition Facts per serving

Calories	458 g
Phosphorus	432 mg
Potassium	207 mg
Sodium	140 mg
Protein	26 g

Carbohydrates   78 g

Lemony Roasted Asparagus
Prep time: 8 minutes
Cook time: 15 minutes
Servings: 4
Ingredients
1 tsp of peel lemon, finely grated
1 tbsp of extra-virgin olive oil
3 tbsp of fresh lemon juice
1 lbs of asparagus spears, (about 18 stems) trimmed
Preparation
1. Heat up the oven to 450 F.
2. Arrange the asparagus on a baking sheet in a single layer.
3. Add lemon peel, oil and lemon juice in a jar. Shake well.
4. Pour mixture on top of the asparagus, stir to coat.
5. Transfer to the oven and roast until tender and crispy, turning once a bit, for about 15 minutes.
6. Best serve warm or at room temperature.

Nutrition Facts per serving
Calories   59 g
Phosphorus   64 mg
Potassium   324 mg
Sodium   2 mg
Protein   2 g
Carbohydrates   6 g

Blasted Garlic Parsnips

Prep time: 10 minutes
Cook time: 20-30 minutes
Servings: 6

Ingredients

3 tbsp of olive oil
1 tbsp of fresh thyme or 1 tsp dry
1/2 sliced large onion
1/4 cup water
8 peeled and sliced garlic cloves
3-4 sliced large parsnips, into 1/4 inch chunks

Preparation

1. Heat up the oven to 350 F.
2. Place the parsnips in a baking dish, add the water and cover with either the lid or use a foil.
3. Bake in the oven for 20-30 minutes.
4. While it's baking, sauté garlic, olive oil, onion and thyme.
5. Add to baking dish and bake until tender, about 20-30 minutes.

Nutrition Facts per serving

Calories	184 g
Phosphorus	117 mg
Potassium	603 mg
Sodium	16 mg
Protein	3 g
Carbohydrates	30 g

Roasted Sweet Onion And Green Beans

Prep time: 5 minutes
Cook time: 45-45 minutes
Servings: 8

Ingredients

2 tbsp of balsamic vinegar
2/3 lbs of green beans
2 tbsp of olive oil
1 lbs of sweet onions, cut into 1/2 size pieces

Preparation

1. Heat up the oven to 375 F.
2. In a large roasting pan, add onions and drizzle with the oil, toss together to evenly coat.
3. Roast in oven for 30 minutes, stirring every 10 minutes.
4. Place the green beans and continue roasting for additional 10 minutes.
5. Pour in the balsamic vinegar and cook about 2 to 5 minutes.

Nutrition Facts per serving

Calories	63 g
Phosphorus	15 mg
Potassium	161 mg
Sodium	6 mg
Protein	1 g
Carbohydrates	7 g

DESSERT RECIPES

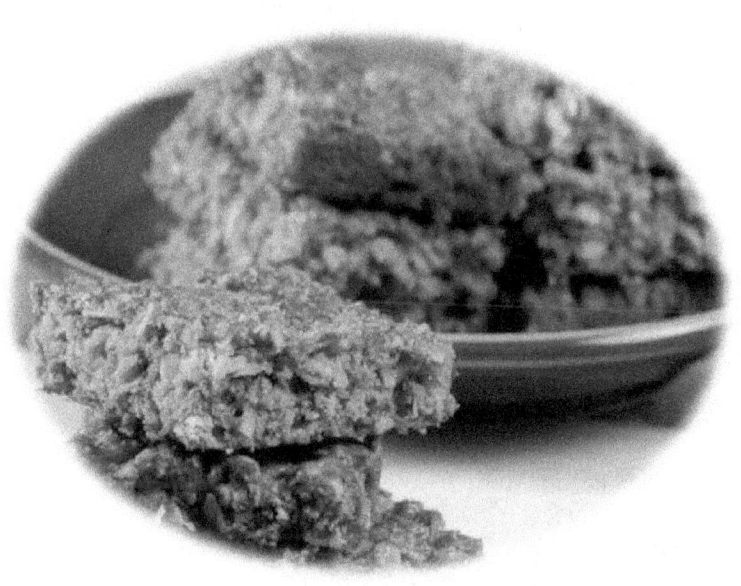

Tibret Sorbet

Servings: 4

Ingredients

Thinly sliced lemon wedge for garnish
1 pasteurized egg white
2 tablespoon of powdered sugar
14 ounces can of litchis or 1 pounds of fresh, peeled and pitted

Preparations

1. Add sugar plus fresh litchi in a food processor or blender and process until smooth.
2. Remove any remaining solids from the puree by Pressing through a fine strainer.

Freeze for about 3 hours.

3. Process the mixture in a processor or a blender until slushy.
4. Add the egg white while the motor is still running
5. Transfer mixture back to the freezer for 8 hours or overnight.
6. Puree mixture on last time in the blender just before serving, top with sliced lemon to garnish.

Nutrition Facts per serving

Calories	95 g
Phosphorus	36 mg
Potassium	207 mg
Sodium	15 mg
Protein	2 g
Carbohydrates	23 g

Blueberry vanilla Bran Muffins

Prep time: 5 minutes
Cook time: 30 minutes
Servings: 24 muffins

Ingredients

1 cup of frozen blueberries, unsweetened
2 cups of plain yogurt
2 teaspoons of baking soda
4 teaspoons of baking powder
2 cups of white flour
2 teaspoons of vanilla extract
2 cups of wheat bran, germ removed
½ cup of oil
2 eggs
1 cup of white sugar

Preparations

1. Mix vanilla, wheat bran, oil, eggs and sugar in a bowl.
2. Mix baking powder and flour together in a separate bowl.
3. Combine yogurt with baking, then mix all the ingredient together.
4. Bake in the oven for 30 minutes at 375 F

Nutrition Facts per serving
Calories	115 g
Phosphorus	109 mg
Potassium	132 mg
Sodium	177 mg
Protein	3.5 g
Carbohydrates	23 g

Blueberry Glazed Citrus Cake Compote

Prep time: 15 minutes
Cook time: 50 to 60 minutes
Servings: 24

Ingredients

Citrus Cake:
1 teaspoon of vanilla
1 teaspoon of orange juice
1 teaspoon of lime juice
1 tablespoon of lemon juice
1 tablespoon of citrus zest (lemon, orange, lime)
3/4 cup of milk
3/4 teaspoon of baking soda
3 cups of all-purpose flour
4 eggs
1 cup of unsalted butter
2 cups of sugar

Glaze:
1 teaspoon of milk
1 teaspoon of orange juice
1 teaspoon of lime juice
1 teaspoon of lemon juice
1 1/2 cup of icing sugar

Blueberry Compote:
4 cups of blueberries
1/2 cup of sugar
1 cup of water

Preparations

For the cake:
1. Heat up the oven to 350 Degrees.
2. Mix sugar and butter in a bowl and add the eggs one by one.
3. Add citrus juice/zest and vanilla. Alternate mixing in the dry ingredient with milk.
4. Pour mixture into 12 cup bundt pan, transfer to the oven and bake for 50 to 60 mins. Set aside a wire rack to cool.

For the glaze:

1. Combine together all ingredients for glaze. Drizzle the cake top with glaze.

For the compote:

1. Combine sugar and water to dissolve over medium heat.
2. Add the blueberries and cook until it reach your desired consistency.

Nutrition Facts per serving
Calories   280 g
Phosphorus   43 mg
Potassium   67 mg
Sodium   56 mg
Protein   4 g
Carbohydrates   47 g

Roasted pear With Honey

Prep time: 5 minutes
Cook time: 30 minutes
Servings: 8

Ingredients

1 teaspoon of vanilla extract
1 teaspoon of lemon zest
1 teaspoon of orange zest
1/2 teaspoon of 5-spice powder
1/4 cup of honey
1/4 cup of lemon juice
1/4 cup of melted margarine
4 pears, remove the skin, halved and cored

Preparations

1. Heat up the oven to 350 Degrees.
2. Add pears into the lemon juice, toss both together to prevent discoloration.
3. In a mixing bowl, combine melted margarine, zest, vanilla, spices and liquid honey and add to pears.
4. Place pears mixture in an oven-safe pan and roast until pears become soft, for 30 minutes. While the pears still retains their shape.

Nutrition Facts per serving
Calories   141 g
Phosphorus   12 mg
Potassium   121 mg
Sodium   2 mg
Protein   0.5 g
Carbohydrates   23 g

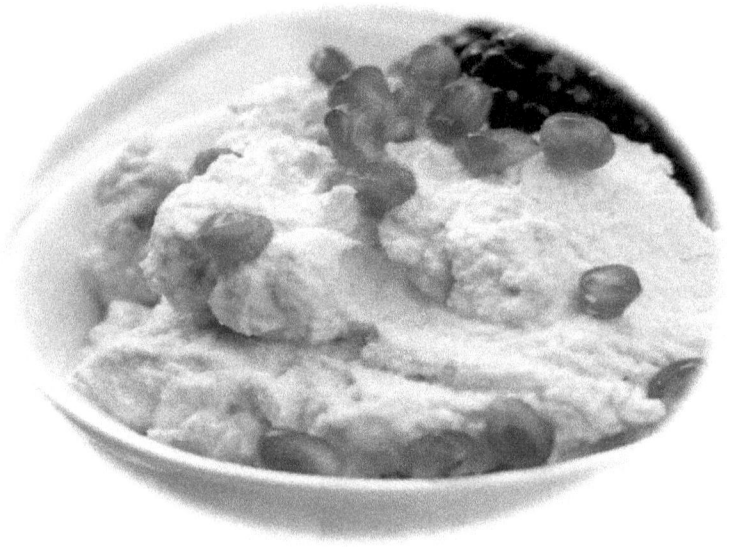

Apple Caramel Pound Cake
Prep time: 10 minutes
Cook time: 50 minutes
Servings: 12
Ingredients
1 box yellow cake mix or any sugar free cake mix
3/4 cup of flour
1/4 cup of caramel flavored syrup, sugar free or regular
3 medium apples, (Granny Smith) peeled, cored and diced
1/4 cup of vegetable oil
2 tbsp of water
12 egg whites

Preparation
1. Warm up the oven to 350 F.
2. Arrange the diced apples in the microwave on high for 6 minutes or until apples are soft. Mash to make applesauce and allow cooling on room temperature.
3. Mix together the flour, caramel flavoring, cake mix, apple mixture, vegetable oil, egg whites and water in a mixing bowl. Mix for 1 minute on low speed, scraping down the sides as you mix. Then Mix once more on medium speed for two minutes.
4. Transfer the batter into a 9 X 13 baking dish or two greased loaf pans.
5. Place in the oven and bake for 30-45 minutes or until a toothpick inserted in the center comes out dry.
6. Once the cake is cool, sprinkle with powdered sugar.

Nutrition Facts per serving
Calories	300 g
Phosphorus	160 mg
Potassium	141 mg
Sodium	319 mg
Protein	7g
Carbohydrates	52 g

Simple Lemon Curd
Servings: 16
Ingredients
1/2 cup of melted butter
3 lemons zest
2/3 cup of fresh lemon juice
3 eggs
1 cup of granulated sugar
Preparation
1. Whisk together the eggs and sugar in a microwave-safe bowl, until smooth.
2. Stir in the butter, lemon zest with juice.

3. Microwave, stirring every one minute until you have a thick mixture, enough to stick to the back of a metal spoon.
4. Transfer the Lemon Curd into small sterile jars.
5. Store in the refrigerator for up to three weeks.

Nutrition Facts per serving
Calories   115 g
Phosphorus   20 mg
Potassium   28 mg
Sodium   54 mg
Protein   1g
Carbohydrates 14 g

Peach with Whipped Cream And Lemon
Servings: 4
Ingredients
8 thinly slices rustic or artisan bread
1/4 tsp of ground cinnamon
4 canned peach halves, finely chopped
3 tsp of olive oil, divided
1/2 tsp of lemon zest
1 tbsp of granulated sugar
1 cup of whipping cream
Preparation
1. Whisk the lemon zest, sugar, and whipping cream, with a wire whisk or an electric mixer until it forms soft peaks.
2. In a medium pan over medium heat, heat 1 teaspoon of olive oil, add peaches and cook for 5-6 minutes.
3. Stir in ground cinnamon.
4. Spread the remaining 2 teaspoons of oil over bread slices.
5. Place in the oven and toast on broil.
6. Top toasted bread slices with peaches mixture and whipped cream.

Nutrition Facts per serving
Calories   190 g
Phosphorus   53 mg
Potassium   127 mg

Sodium   203 mg
Protein   4g
Carbohydrates 25 g

Molded Popcorn Balls

Servings: 18

Ingredients

18 cups of air popped popcorn, (about 8 1/2 tbsp of non-popped popcorn kernels)
1 tsp of vanilla
2 cups of sugar
1 tsp of vinegar
1/2 cup of light corn syrup
1 1/2 cups of water
Butter for coating

Preparation

1. Coat the sides of a medium stock pan with butter.
2. Heat water, sugar, vinegar and syrup over medium heat, stirring constantly until sugar is dissolved. Bring to a boil.
3. Keep boiling, stirring occasionally until sauce temperature gets to 250 F (hard ball candy stage). Turn heat off and stir in vanilla.
4. Pour the syrup over popcorn in a large bowl, stirring until finely coated.
5. Let mixture stand until cool enough to handle.
6. Coat your hands with butter and mold popcorn into 2 1/2 inch balls.

Nutrition Facts per serving
Calories   146 g
Phosphorus   29 mg
Potassium   27 mg
Sodium   7 mg
Protein   1g
Carbohydrates   36 g

Pumpkin Spice Mousse Pie

Servings: 8

Ingredients

1 baked pie shell, cooled
3 1/2 cups of nondairy whipped topping (Cool Whip)
1 tsp of pumpkin spice or 1/2 tsp each of nutmeg, ginger, and cinnamon
1/2 cup of canned pumpkin
1 small package instant vanilla pudding
3/4 cup of milk

Preparation

1. Combine pudding mix with milk and beat for 2 minutes or until it becomes thick.
2. Mix in pumpkin pie spice and pumpkin.
3. Slowly mix in two cups of Cool Whip into the mixture and pour into pie shell.
4. Place in the Refrigerator for about 4 hours.
5. Lastly add the remaining Cool Whip to the top.

Nutrition Facts per serving

Calories	238 g
Phosphorus	128 mg
Potassium	110 mg
Sodium	294 mg
Protein	2g
Carbohydrates	30 g

Crocked Pot Pina Cherry Cake

Servings: 8-10

Ingredients

1/2 cup of unsalted butter, diced
Sprinkle of cinnamon
1 package of yellow cake mix
1 (20 oz) can of lite cherry pie filling
1 (20 oz) can of crushed pineapple

Preparation

1. Grease the crock pot's sides and bottom very well.
2. Spread layer in this order: pineapple, pie filling, and the cake mix. Top with a sprinkle of cinnamon and layer dices butter over the cake mix.
3. Cover with the lid and Cook for 2 to 3 hours on high.

Nutrition Facts per serving

Calories	459 g
Phosphorus	222 mg
Potassium	230 mg
Sodium	441 mg
Protein	4g
Carbohydrates	70 g

SIDE AND SNACKS

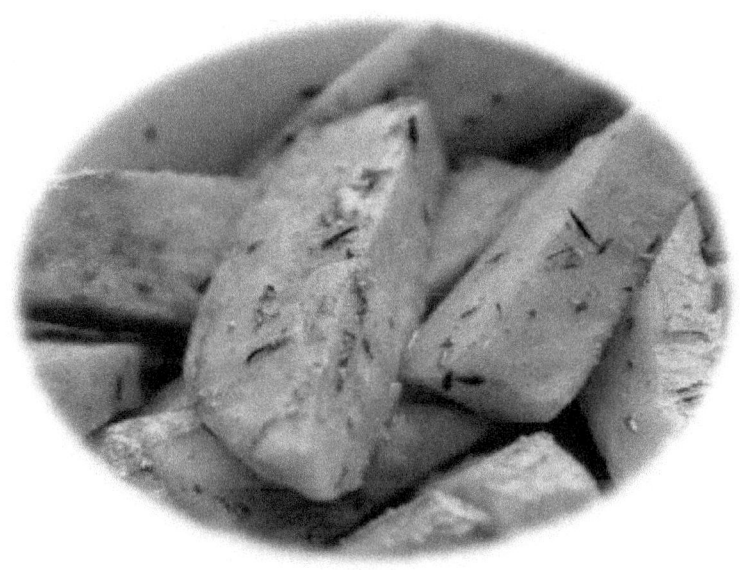

Orange Chocolate Cookies
Prep time: 10 minutes
Cook time: 10 minutes
Servings: 36
Ingredients
2 cups of raisins
2/3 cup of orange juice
4 eggs
1/4 cup of powdered artificial sweetener
1 1/3 cups of margarine

1 tbsp of low sodium baking powder
1 cup of cocoa powder, unsweetened
3 cups of all-purpose flour
Preparation
1. Heat up the oven to 375 F.
2. Sift together baking powder, flour and cocoa.
3. Beat margarine with a hand or stand mixer until creamy; beat in sweetener.
4. Beat in the eggs until smooth.
5. Alternatively, add orange juice with the dry ingredients. Stir in raisins.
6. Place the dough in teaspoon measure on the baking sheets. (Do no grease)
7. Bake in the oven for 10 minutes. Remove cookies and allow to cool.

Nutrition Facts per serving
Calories   141 g
Phosphorus   52 mg
Potassium   139 mg
Sodium   66 mg
Protein   2g
Carbohydrates   17 g

Honey Cornmeal Muffins
Prep time: 10 minutes
Cook time: 20-25 minutes
Servings: 12
Ingredients
1/2 cup of no added salt canned corn
1/2 cup of buttermilk
1/4 cup of honey
2 eggs
1/2 cup of softened butter, unsalted
1/4 cup of granulated sugar
1/2 tsp of baking soda
1 cup of cornmeal

1 cup of all-purpose flour

Preparation

1. Preheat oven to 400 F.
2. Grease muffin pan lightly with cooking oil spray.
3. Combine baking soda, flour, sugar and cornmeal in a large bowl.
4. Use either a food processor or pastry blender to mix in the butter until butter is pea-sized.
5. Beat eggs in a different bowl, mix in buttermilk and honey.
6. Pour the buttermilk/egg mixture into the dry ingredients, stirring until just combined.
7. Slowly mix in the corn. Place batter in muffin cups and bake in the oven for 20-25 minutes or until it becomes dry when a skewer is inserted into the middle of the muffin.

Nutrition Facts per serving
Calories   203 g
Phosphorus   67 mg
Potassium   89 mg
Sodium   79 mg
Protein   4 g
Carbohydrates   28 g

Dilled Vinegar Carrots

Prep time: 7 minutes
Cook time: 3-5 minutes
Servings: 6

Ingredients

2 tsp of garlic powder or fresh garlic
1/4 tsp of pepper
3 tbsp of sugar
2 tsp of dill weed
1/2 cup of plain rice vinegar
1 1/2 cups of white vinegar
1 lbs of carrots, cut into small strips

Preparation
1. Steam carrot strips in microwave for 3-5 minutes.
2. Plunge the carrots into ice water to cool.
3. Mix together the rest ingredients and spread on carrots.
4. Transfer in an airtight container, cover and chill overnight.

Nutrition Facts per serving
Calories   58 g
Phosphorus   28 mg
Potassium   246 mg
Sodium   56 mg
Protein   1 g
Carbohydrates   14 g

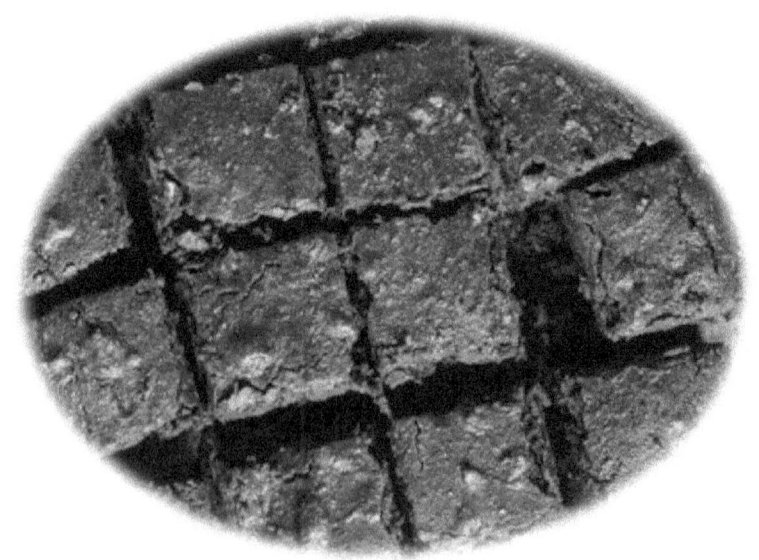

Dried Cranberries With Green Beans Hazelnuts

Prep time: 10 minutes
Cook time: 25 minutes
Servings: 8

Ingredients

1/2 tsp of lemon zest
1/2 cup of dried cranberries
1/3 cup of thinly sliced shallots
3 tbsp of olive oil
12 cups of water
1/2 cup of hazelnuts
1 1/2 lbs of green beans (fresh or frozen)

Preparation

1. Heat up the oven to 350 F.
2. In a single layer, spread the hazelnuts on a baking sheet. Bake in the oven for 10-15 minutes at 350 degrees or until skins is starting to split, turning once.
3. Arrange the toasted hazelnuts to a dish or colander, and use a towel to rub briskly to remove the skins. Chop nuts coarsely.
4. Boil water (12 cups) in a large saucepan. Add beans and cook until tender and crisp, about 4 minutes. Drain and cool by plunging into ice water, drain again and Pat dry.
5. Heat oil over medium heat in a large skillet, swirl to coat. Cook shallots in the skillet until shallots are lightly browned.
6. Add in the beans, cook until heated thoroughly, about 3 minutes, stirring not too frequent. Add hazelnuts and cranberries, cook additional 1 minute. Top with sprinkle of lemon zest.

Nutrition Facts per serving

Calories	199 g
Phosphorus	73 mg
Potassium	246 mg
Sodium	19 mg
Protein	4 g
Carbohydrates	17 g

Toasted bread with Goat Cheese And Green Tomatoes

Prep time: 7 minutes
Cook time: 7-8 minutes
Servings: 4

Ingredients

8 toasted slices of French bread
Ground pepper to taste
4 tsp of olive oil
1 cup of crumbled goat cheese,
2 tsp of minced oregano leaves
1 tbsp of balsamic vinegar
4 medium green tomatoes, cut in 1/2 inch thick slices

Preparation

1. Coat oil on the inside of a shallow baking dish.
2. Layer slices of tomato in the bottom of the dish in a single overlapping layer.
3. Sprinkle vinegar over the tomatoes and spread minced oregano on top of tomatoes.
4. Add goat cheese to the top and then drizzle with olive oil.
5. Preheat the oven broiler, place the tomatoes 5-8 inches underneath the broiler,
broil about 7-8 minutes or cheese is just beginning to brown and tomatoes are hot.
6. Arrange over toasted slices of bread, add pepper to taste.

Nutrition Facts per serving

Calories	173 g
Phosphorus	161 mg
Potassium	280 mg
Sodium	135 mg
Protein	7 g
Carbohydrates	9 g

Mixed Bread Pudding

Prep time: 10 minutes
Cook time: 50 minutes
Servings: 10

Ingredients

Whipped cream
½ tsp of cinnamon
1 tbsp of orange zest
2 tsp of vanilla
½ cup of sugar
12-oz bag of frozen berry medley, thawed
2 cups of heavy cream
6 eggs, beaten
8 cups cubed challah bread

Preparation

1. Heat up the oven to 375° Degrees.
2. Beat sugar, eggs cream, cinnamon, vanilla and orange zest in a bowl until smooth.
3. Mix in fruit and bread cubes with hands.
4. Grease a baking pan and pour mixture into the pan. Bake in the oven for 35 minutes, covered in foil.
5. Remove the foil and continue baking for 15 more minutes. Let sit for 10 minutes in oven.
6. Cut bread pudding and top with whipped cream.

Nutrition Facts per serving

Calories	392 g
Phosphorus	134 mg
Potassium	172 mg
Sodium	321 mg
Protein	9 g
Carbohydrates	36 g

Simple Chipotle Wings

Prep time: 10 minutes
Cook time: 18-20 minutes
Servings: 4

Ingredients

1 tbsp of chopped chives
1 tsp of black pepper
¼ cup of slightly melted butter, unsalted
¼ cup of honey
1½ tbsp of diced chipotle peppers in adobo sauce
Oil for greasing baking pan
1 lbs of fresh jumbo chicken wings, cut into pieces

Preparation

1. Preheat oven to 400° Degrees.
2. Add the chicken wings pieces onto a greased baking pan.
3. Bake in the oven, turning halfway through the cooking time for 18–20 minutes, or until crispy and the internal temperature on an instant-read thermometer reads 165° F.
4. In a large bowl, mix the rest ingredients using a rubber spatula, until totally combined.
5. Withdraw baked chicken wings from the oven, add into the bowl containing sauce and toss until coated evenly.

Nutrition Facts per serving

Calories	384 g
Phosphorus	146 mg
Potassium	266 mg
Sodium	99 mg
Protein	20 g
Carbohydrates	18 g

Pineapple cabbage Coleslaw

Servings: 4

Ingredients

(Optional) Dash of pepper
1/4 cup of Miracle Whip
1/4 cup of chopped onion
1 (8 oz) can of crushed unsweetened pineapple, drained
2 cups of shredded cabbage

Preparation

1. Mix together all the Pineapple Coleslaw ingredients in a bowl.
2. Chill in the refrigerator at least 1 hour before serving.

Nutrition Facts per serving

Calories	72 g
Phosphorus	15 mg
Potassium	153 mg
Sodium	137 mg
Protein	1g
Carbohydrates	11 g

Refreshing Energy Bars

Prep Time: 15 minutes
Cook Time: 40 minutes
Servings: 8 servings per recipe

Ingredients

1/3 cup of applesauce
1/3 cup of shredded coconut
3 tbsp of honey
1/4 cup of semi-sweet mini chocolate chips
1 cup of rolled oats
3 tbsp of unsalted chopped peanuts
3 large eggs
1/2 tsp of ground cinnamon

Preparation

1. Warm-up the oven to 325F. Coat cooking spray over a 9×9 inch pan.
2. Combine together the coconut, oats, chocolate chips, peanuts, and cinnamon in a mixing bowl.
3. In a small bowl, beat together the eggs, add honey and applesauce and stir well.
4. Combine the wet mixture into the dry mix, stir until finely combine.
5. Spread mixture into the base of the prepared pan. Press evenly.
6. Arrange in the heated oven and cook for 40 minutes. When it's done, allow to cool before cutting into bars.

Can keep in an airtight container in the refrigerator for up to a week.

Nutrition Facts per serving
Calories	206 g
Phosphorus	163 mg
Potassium	182 mg
Sodium	35 mg
Dietary Fiber	8 g
Protein	7 g
Carbohydrates	27 g

STAPLES

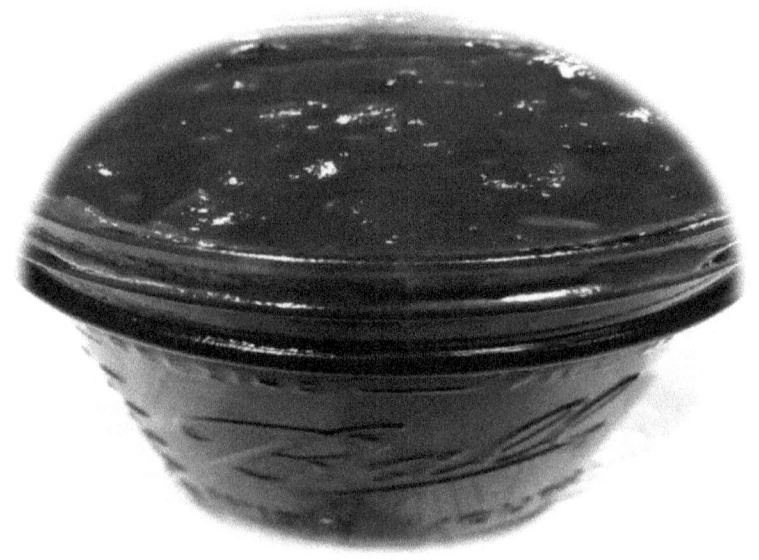

All Purpose Herb Blend

Servings: 2 tablespoons servings

Ingredients

1 tbsp of celery seed
1 tbsp of dill weed
1 tbsp of dried oregano
2 tbsp of dried tarragon
1/4 cup of dried parsley

Preparation

1. Mix together all the ingredients and store in an air-tight container up to 1 year.

Nutrition Facts per serving
Calories   tbd
Phosphorus   0 mg
Potassium   0 mg
Sodium   0 mg
Protein   0 g
Carbohydrates   0 g

Cajun Seasoning

Servings: 2

Ingredients

2 teaspoon of paprika
2 teaspoon of onion powder
2 teaspoon of garlic powder
1 teaspoon of cayenne or 2 teaspoons for medium spice

Preparation

1. Mix together all the ingredients in a mixing bowl. Store in an air-tight container.

Nutrition Facts per serving
Calories   25 g
Phosphorus   5 mg

Potassium   36 mg
Sodium   15 mg
Protein   1 g
Carbohydrates   5 g

Basil Garlic-Herb Seasoning

Ingredients:

1 tsp of powdered lemon rind
1 tsp of Oregano
1 tsp of Basil
2 tsp of Garlic powder

Preparation

1. Use a blender to mix the ingredients together. Store with a few grains of rice in an air-tight container to keep it from clumping.

Nutrition Facts per serving
Calories   12 g
Phosphorus   16 mg
Potassium   47 mg
Sodium   1 mg
Protein   0 g
Carbohydrates   3 g

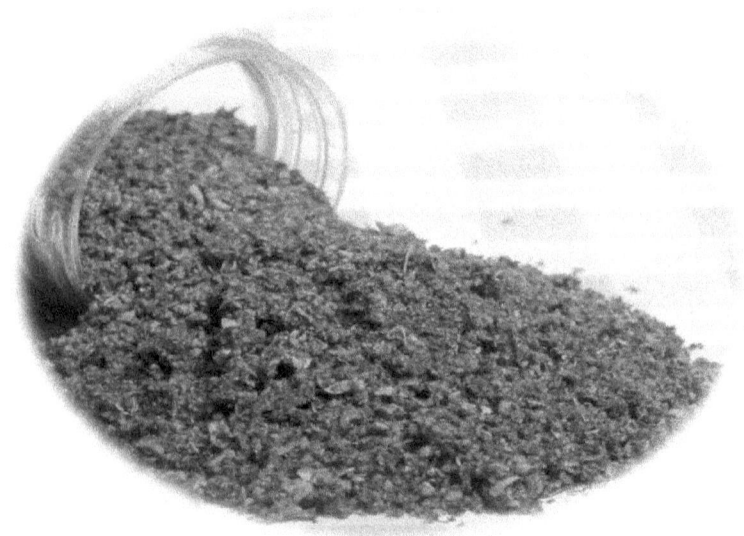

Simple Low Sodium Soy Sauce

Servings: 32

Ingredients

2 tbsp of Kikkoman Low Sodium Soy Sauce
1/4 tsp of garlic powder
1/4 tsp of powdered ginger
1/4 tsp of black pepper
2 cups of boiling water
4-5 tbsp of molasses
6 tbsp of cider or balsamic vinegar
5 packets of Low Sodium Herb-ox Bouillon, chicken or beef flavor

Preparation

1. Mix together all the ingredients in a mixing bowl.

Transfer into bottle and store indefinitely in the refrigerator.

Nutrition Facts per serving
Calories   trace
Phosphorus   15 mg
Potassium   30 mg
Sodium   70 mg
Protein   trace
Carbohydrates trace

Sarah's BBQ Sauce

Servings: 6

Ingredients

1/8 tsp of ground black pepper
1/2 tsp of onion powder
1/2 tsp of garlic powder
3/4 cup of no-salt added ketchup
2 tbsp of mustard
2 tbsp of canola oil
1/4 cup of rice wine (or other white) vinegar
1/4 cup of low sodium soy sauce
1/4 cup of Worcestershire sauce
3/4 cup of brown sugar

Preparation

1. Whisk all ingredients together until well blended. Use right away or refrigerate for up to 2 weeks.

Nutrition Facts per serving

Calories	46 g
Phosphorus	8 mg
Potassium	56 mg
Sodium	102 mg
Protein	0
Carbohydrates	8

Easy Poultry Seasoning

Servings: 11

Ingredients

1 tsp of ground black pepper
2 tsp of dried marjoram
2 tsp of dried thyme
2 tbsp of dried ground sage

Preparation

1. Mix together all the ingredients in a mixing bowl. Store in an air tight container up to a year.

Nutrition Facts per serving

Calories	3 g
Phosphorus	1 mg
Potassium	8 mg
Sodium	0 mg
Protein	0
Carbohydrates	8 g

Mustard Red Chili Vinegar

Servings: 8, 2 tablespoons each

Ingredients

1/2 cup of olive oil
1 tbsp of chili powder
Pepper to taste
1/4 cup of red wine vinegar
1 tbsp of chopped shallots
2 tbsp of dijon mustard

Preparation

1. Whisk vinegar, chili powder, pepper, shallots and mustard together in a bowl.
2. Whisk the olive oil in slowly until emulsified. Adjust taste by adding chili powder.

Nutrition Facts per serving

Calories 134 g
Phosphorus   4 mg
Potassium   31 mg
Sodium   40 mg
Protein   1
Carbohydrates 2 g

Mixed Mexican Blend

Servings: 2 tablespoons

Ingredients

1 tbsp of onion powder
1/2 tsp of cinnamon
1/4 cup of chili powder
1 tsp of garlic powder
1 tsp of dried oregano
1 tsp of crushed red pepper
1 tbsp of ground cumin

Preparation

1. Combine together all the ingredients in a bowl and store in an air-tight container up to a year.

Fajita Flavored Marinade

Servings: 15

Ingredients

3 tbsp of vegetable oil
2 crushed garlic cloves, or 1/4 teaspoon dried
1 finely diced jalapeño
2 limes juice
1 grapefruit juice
1 orange juice

Preparation

1. In a small mixing bowl, mix together all the ingredients.
2. Use marinate for all sort of poultry, fish, meat etc. for at least an hour before barbequing pan-frying or grilling.

Nutrition Facts per serving

Calories 33 g
Phosphorus 5 mg
Potassium 42 mg
Sodium 0 mg
Protein 0 g
Carbohydrates 2 g

Homemade Mushroom Broth

Cook time: 10 minus
Servings: 2-4

Ingredients

1/2 cup of chopped carrots and celery
5-8 mushrooms, dried
1/2 cup of chopped onions
2-4 cups of water

Preparation

1. Combine together all the ingredients in a saucepan, heat until it boils, reduce heat and simmer for 10 minutes.
2. Turn the heat off and strain.

Nutrition Facts per serving
Calories 24 g
Carbohydrates 4 g
Potassium 62 mg
Phosphorus 8 mg
Protein 1g
Sodium 20 mg

Common Measuring units

1 lbs = 453 g

1 oz=30g

½ oz= 15g

2 oz= 60g

6 ½ oz (195 g)

1/8 tsp =½ mL

1/2 tsp =2.5 mL

½ tsp =2 mL

1 tsp =5 mL

½ tbsp=7.5ml

1 tbsp =15 mL

2 tbsp = 30 mL

⅔ lb =300 g

¼ cup =60 mL

½ cup =125 mL

1 cup = 250ml

2 cups=500ml

3 cups =750 mL

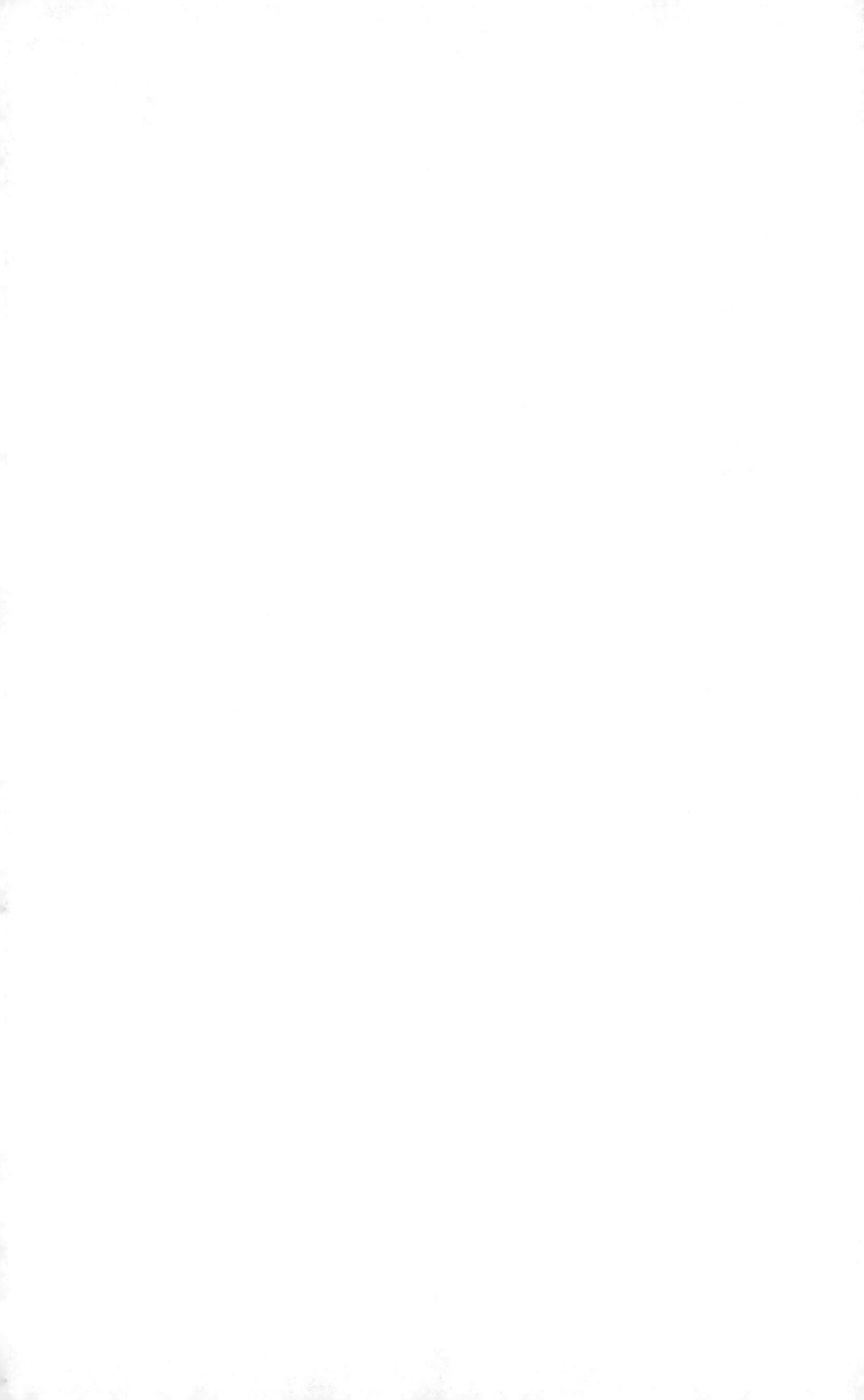

CPSIA information can be obtained
at www.ICGtesting.com
Printed in the USA
LVHW011515280621
691349LV00012B/789